A NEW LIFE

Other Bantam Books of interest
Ask your bookseller for the books you have missed

BETTER HOMES & GARDENS NEW BABY BOOK
COMPLETE BOOK OF BREASTFEEDING
  by Marvin S. Eiger, M.D. and Sally Wendkos Olds
NAME YOUR BABY by Lareina Rule
UNDERSTANDING PREGNANCY AND CHILDCARE
  by Sheldon H. Cherry, M.D.
FEED ME! I'M YOURS by Vicki Lansky
FIRST TWELVE MONTHS OF LIFE by Frank Caplan

A NEW LIFE

Martha Vanceburg

BANTAM BOOKS
NEW YORK · TORONTO · LONDON · SYDNEY · AUCKLAND

For Marty, and for David, Jennifer, and Molly, with special thanks to Amy, Anita, Anna, Elizabeth, Ginger, Joan, Jolene, Lisa, Lucy, Marcia, Mary Ray, Nancy, Pat A., Pat D., and Patricia, and of course to Howard M. Levine, M.D., and John J. Sciarra, M.D., Ph.D.

A NEW LIFE
A Bantam Book / June 1990

Library of Congress Cataloging-in-Publication Data

Vanceburg, Martha,
    A new life / Martha Vanceburg.
      p.   cm.
    ISBN 0-553-34882-5
    1. Pregnancy—Miscellanea.   I Title.
RG525.V33   1990
616.2'4—dc20   90-230
                                              CIP

ACKNOWLEDGMENTS

Grateful acknowledgment is made for permission to reprint previously published material. For copyright notices, see the Acknowledgments section on pages iv–viii, which constitutes an extension of the copyright page.

Published simultaneously in the United States and Canada

Bantam Books are published by Bantam Books, a division of Bantam Doubleday Dell Publishing Group, Inc. Its trademark, consisting of the words "Bantam Books" and the portrayal of a rooster, is Registered in U.S. Patent and Trademark Office and in other countries. Marca Registrada. Bantam Books, 666 Fifth Avenue, New York, New York 10103.

PRINTED IN THE UNITED STATES OF AMERICA

FFG   0 9 8 7 6 5 4 3 2 1

A NEW LIFE

Day 1

He embraced me and now I am someone else; someone else in the pulse that repeats in the pulse of my own veins and in the breath that mingles with my breath. Now my belly is as noble as my heart.

—GABRIELA MISTRAL

This is the day on which your life begins to change, as profoundly as possible. All your life, you have been one person, now you're going to be two. If you find this an odd, wonderful, disconcerting feeling—joyful yet a little frightening at the same time—you can rest assured that most women do.

As people have no doubt already told you, ambivalence is perfectly normal. You may feel like an empress one moment and like a character in a horror movie the next. Even with this ambivalence, many women feel a new sense of spiritual connection at this time—a deep, warm bond with the source of all love and healing.

Whatever you are feeling, it's bound to be new and strange. Many books, relatives, friends, and your doctor or other birth advisors can give you factual information, but you may feel the need to renew your spiritual consciousness. These pages will accompany you on the journey you've begun, with running commentary on the emotional, as well as physical changes you'll be going through; your body isn't the only aspect of you that's undergoing profound changes.

THOUGHT FOR TODAY: Whatever I'm feeling, I was meant to feel it. I'm right on track, and so is my baby, for our great adventure.

Day 2

Let the soul be a swimming animal.
Let it scrape the bottom. Breathe
Water until it grows gills.
— FRANCES MAYES

Perhaps if we lived in a culture that focused more attention on women and children, birthing and growing, the subtle signs of this new life's progress would be more intelligible. But our world doesn't make much room for pregnancy and birth, so each pregnant woman must make her own.

Today the embryo's cells continue to double every few hours—thirty-two; sixty-four; a hundred and twenty-eight. Probably the little clump of cells has made its way through one of your tubes toward your uterus. You'll never know which side it chose. The new life already has its directions programmed inside, just as a flower seed knows to send its roots down and its stalk up.

Remember that you have company on this journey. Not only the unknown friend suspended deep inside you; you also have a spiritual guide, the source of your most powerful longings and rewards. The path to motherhood—from being one fertile body to being two separate people—is a proud and well-traveled one, yet each mother makes her journey alone. What will yours hold? After the birth your body will gradually return to what it was, but an expanded spirit can be yours forever.

THOUGHT FOR TODAY: No matter what cultural messages I receive, I am proud and honored to be pregnant.

Day 3

Love set you going, like a fat gold watch.
—SYLVIA PLATH

It would be nice to think that you and your partner made love with the baby in mind, and your love for each other deepened when you realized you could be making a new life. But its growth will proceed with no conscious help from you—without your knowledge or maybe even awareness.

Today may be the day your embryo attaches itself to the wall of your uterus, like a small mammal beginning hibernation. Your body will gradually stretch to accommodate it, and so will your spirit. It will grow as a bud grows, first small and secretly and then more openly—disclosing new richness.

Whether you made your baby deliberately or not, its growth is part of your body now. You are both your own old self and a new one, a watch-pocket, a secret holder for a precious new design.

THOUGHT FOR TODAY. I feel blessed with the secret knowledge of what's budding inside me, and I'll pray for patience during the long months before my pocket opens.

Day 4

> *Life is but an endless series of experiments.*
> —M.K. GANDHI

You still can't really feel it—or can you?—but your pregnancy is progressing as it should. Your body makes the necessary adjustments; preparing to increase your circulation, the volume of your blood increases (it has to nourish two of you, now) as well as your many yards of blood vessels. Your spirit prepares as well. You may find your focus turning increasingly inward. Your new life is a child of your spirit as well as of your body. Along with essential nutrients from the foods you eat, you can surround it with serenity and love.

So far, the new life is a successful experiment, and you and it are partners in life's greatest adventure. The early hours and days of this pregnancy are full of dangers for a new little life; many don't make it this far, but yours did, cushioned in its deluxe laboratory. You could decide to treat this whole pregnancy as an experiment in trying to make yourself the best mother you can: playing music for your baby, singing to it, taking it swimming and walking and speaking to it of the wonders that lie in store.

THOUGHT FOR TODAY: Perhaps I can use this experimental attitude to teach myself how to live better. I will try to learn to love what's best for me, in food, spiritual nourishment—in all aspects of my life.

Day 5

> *Think of the whole haystack—*
> *a composition so fortuitous*
> *it only looks monumental.*
> *There's always a straw twitching somewhere.*
> —ADRIENNE RICH

Of course you would like this pregnancy to be perfect. You probably want to have the perfect, classic outline of a pregnant woman; to have just so much morning sickness and fatigue, and no more; to have cravings and mood swings in correct proportion, at the correct time; and to give birth to the perfect, classic baby on the exact date your doctor calculated.

Because you haven't done this before, you don't know exactly what to expect. So you think of images from books, movies, and TV, although you understand at least with part of your mind that you're not acting in a scripted comedy-drama. This is your real life, and your pregnancy is part of you, not some sitcom. If you're the kind of person who takes things seriously, you'll take this very seriously; if you're pretty easygoing, you'll take this more casually.

Either way, you can seize this opportunity to deepen your spiritual connection to whatever source of love powers your personal world. However you think of this life power, it can comfort and sustain you.

THOUGHT FOR TODAY: For me, pregnancy will be an opportunity to deepen my self-knowledge and to grow spiritually. I know perfection is impossible, but I want to do the best I can.

Day 6

How shall I find a shelter in the clouds, driven by
gods, gold breaking out of them everywhere?
Nothing is what it pretends.
                                        —MADELINE DE FREES

All day you walk around with this secret inside you, delighted, scared, worried, proud. What will this pregnancy do to your body—to your sexuality? How will it change the rest of your life? How will you change? It's very hard to surrender to the unknown.

Already your unseen guest has been responsible for changes that are hard to define. Some women have moments of such fatigue they feel they could fall asleep standing up. Many feel queasy and nauseous, and no matter what they eat or drink, nothing seems to agree with them.

Some people say, "You'll lose your taste for coffee"; "You won't want to eat spicy foods"; "You'll crave ice cream." Others say that from the moment of conception, they didn't want to eat anything at all, while still other women report being ravenously hungry for nine solid months.

Besides nourishing your body, you can nourish your spirit. Through prayer and meditation, you can deepen your channel of communication with a power greater than yourself. Your body is engaged in the great work of building another body; your spirit must be busy, too.

THOUGHT FOR TODAY: I need more than one kind of nourishment.

Day 7

Observe the tall cold of a Flower
which is as innocent and as guilty,
as meaningful and as meaningless as any
other flower in the western field.
—GWENDOLYN BROOKS

In a week or ten days you can have the test that will tell you definitively whether or not you're pregnant. Some women believe they know before any test results; they feel as though another life had started within them, as though they've begun a long, irreversible process that will create a mother and a new family.

You look the same as you did eight days ago. What line have you crossed? When I was a teenager, we used to joke that there's no such thing as being slightly pregnant. Things are happening in your hypothalamus, your pituitary, the hormone-secreting centers in your brain; a new ball of cells has imbedded itself in the wall of your uterus. These new realities use a lot of energy.

Now is the time to begin your surrender to this process, and the first step may be accepting that you don't know anything for sure. You still don't know for certain whether or not you really are pregnant; if you are, you don't know who will be born or what kind of a mother you will be. This is a lot to take on trust, yet trust is all you have for sure.

THOUGHT FOR TODAY: I trust in a benign destiny for me and my baby.

When was this to be?
The first leaves of the
cutback hydrangea

are opening. The earth
is like a fist
threatening nothing.
——Cid Corman

In the days and weeks to come, you'll unfold along with your baby, and your spirit will learn a new language of loving and relatedness. Sometimes women report that their conscious thoughts obsess about What Might Happen to them, to their babies, to our frail, shared world. Disasters, illnesses, wars seem much closer and more threatening than they did before. Yet much more is going right in your life than wrong.

We are held to life by a power greater than ourselves. Your pregnancy is part of the fulfillment of that plan, and whatever happens was meant to happen. You can choose to surrender joyously, doing your best to see that your child gets the best care possible and leaving the rest up to a higher power. Or, you may decide to go on with your life as though nothing special had happened. You may even want to set aside some time every day, or as often as you can, to meditate on the mysteries unfolding. Whatever you choose, remember you are part of a larger plan that is revealing itself exactly as it should.

THOUGHT FOR TODAY: I can choose how to expend whatever energy I have, and I choose to rejoice.

Day 9

Welcome, precious stone of the night,
Delight of the skies, precious stone of the night,
Mother of stars, precious stone of the night,
Child reared by the sun, precious stone of the night. . . .
—GAELIC WELCOME TO THE MOON

Besides being your child, the baby you carry is a child of the universe, like you, and carrying it can give you a deeper connection between your individual life and consciousness and the world's. You are in the hands of the same spirit that sustains all life. Your conscious concerns have been launched forward in time, because your child's life will be led in the future.

Whatever the future holds, it is influenced by the actions we take in the present. Your sense of the connectedness of life can be strengthened by your bond with the new life. You could imagine your child as a beam of light that projects your heart and mind into future time and space.

In this way, the presence of the baby augments your spirit. You can feel the shadow of its hand within your hand, its heartbeat within your own. It doubles your power and also your responsibilities.

THOUGHT FOR TODAY: Sometimes the mystery of my child's existence confuses me, but the joy of its presence gives me greater peace and awareness.

Day 10

In a single instant, a tiny spark can be fanned into a blaze.
—Pedro Calderón de la Barca

Some women believe that, looking back, they can identify the moment of conception. How amazing, this joining of a male and a female cell . . . in virtual silence. Yet it's the beginning of everything.

Your life began this way, as did mine, our parents' lives, and all our mothers and fathers before. The tiny spark inside you is growing, powered by the force that drives all living things, whales and pussy willow buds, the yeast in bread dough, mollusks and beetles and condors. What began in an instant has changed your body and your whole life.

However many times this happens, the microscopic miracle that started it is always amazing—one fertilized cell splitting in two, then in four, eight, sixteen. Probably you'll never know the exact timing; the body's secrets can't always be known. But faith and hope can bring you acceptance and a sense of clarity.

THOUGHT FOR TODAY: I am given over to this process now, and even though I'm sometimes a little scared by its vast impersonality, I'm also deeply glad to join in the work of creation.

Day 11

I, like the zucchini, had been growing since early spring, was tending my crop through the warm months to be delivered in the late, dark part of the year.

—ROBERTA ISRAELOFF

The great wheel of the seasons will swing around three-quarters of a year during your pregnancy. Chances are, you'll never have quite the same relation to these months again. If it's hot, you'll remember that pregnancy made you extra hot; if wet or cold or icy, your pregnancy will be part of your sense of all those weathers. One woman described it like this: "Pregnancy has hollowed out an extra space in my consciousness; all of me must expand to nurture and contain my baby."

Graceful and bountiful as a squash vine, you also have the spiritual imagination to observe your pregnancy and participate fully in it. Just as your bodily awareness will permanently transform your sense of the seasons, pregnancy will transform your whole consciousness. If you decide to keep a journal of these days, you can look forward to sharing it with your baby, years from now.

THOUGHT FOR TODAY: Pregnancy has expanded my weathers and my world; every day I will honor this new connection.

Day 12

All that we call beautiful, the shape of a balcony, a certain landscape, a phrase, an alphabet, the curve of an airplane wing, a mathematical formula, is a kind of vessel, like love, that holds what we know.

—Susan Griffin

When your baby is born, it will be both strange and familiar to you—someone known more intimately than you have ever known anyone else, yet someone you have never seen; someone made from your body, yet someone with a future that will probably take it far beyond you.

We know what the phrase "mother and child" means, but most women have occasional doubts about their mothering abilities. We know about mothering from our own mothers. Most of us have a history of some conflict with our mothers while we were growing up, but we come to accept that they did the best they could. More importantly, we can remember what it's like to be a child. If you can summon those memories and use them, they'll ease your anxieties about motherhood.

Your lives are braided together, as yours is with your mother's, and your memories of childhood will guide you in caring for your baby. You will try to spare it some of the rough spots on the road you traveled; but it's bound to surprise you with its individuality.

THOUGHT FOR TODAY: As long as I have trust in the rightness of what I'm doing, we'll be all right.

Day 13

Today's children are the first generation to grow up in a world that has the power to destroy itself.

—MARGARET MEAD

Unhappily, these words were written a long time ago, and they have been true for several generations. Your baby's generation won't be the first (and we hope it's not the last) to grow up with this knowledge and this power. Even now, when your baby is still more of an idea to you than a reality, you can think about its responsibilities to its fellow creatures and to the world we share.

Peace is too vital to be left in the hands of a small group of soldiers or politicians. Let us hope that in the world your baby inherits, everyone will long for peace, study peace, and understand that nations and peoples have much more in common than not. If you pledge yourself to think peace to your baby while you are joined, and to teach it peace after it is born, the terrible risks of destruction will come to seem unthinkable, and your child's love for this beautiful world will help to keep them far away.

THOUGHT FOR TODAY: I'll teach my child the axiom, "There is no way to peace; peace is the way."

> *To make a prairie takes a clover and one bee,*
> *One clover, and a bee,*
> *And revery—*
> *The revery alone will do,*
> *If bees are few—*
>
> —EMILY DICKINSON

Whether you have ever learned to meditate or not, this is the perfect time to acquire skills in meditation, dreaming, reverie. Your baby is like a dream you carry with you always, since your body is now divided subtly between you.

If you have another child, your need for private space will be even greater. Your child needs your love and loyalty to help in the enormous transition that the new baby will bring to your family, but you must be able to create your own peace and serenity, if you're to be able to spread it around.

Under the sun or the winter sky, on asphalt pavement or in fields of clover, we are all embraced by a protective spirit. And, if invoked through prayer or meditation, it reveals the spark of divinity that dwells within each of us and provides inner peace and serenity.

THOUGHT FOR TODAY: My spiritual legacy to my children will be as important as their physical inheritance. During pregnancy I'll make sure I care for both.

> *Life is nibbling us with little*
> *lips, circling our knees, our*
> *shoulders.*
> *What's the difference,*
> *a kiss or a fin-caress.*
> —DENISE LEVERTOV

Did you imagine it, or are your nipples tingling? It's hard to say how much of what you feel is really due to the physical changes of this pregnancy and how much is imagination, desire to feel something. Some women do, however, feel very real cases of morning queasiness or nausea.

Many have found that leaving some crackers at bedside, nibbling them before you even brush your teeth, can help you to cope with morning nausea. Having a little something in your stomach seems to settle it, although the smell of coffee may not be as welcome as usual.

It may seem very odd to have your habits disrupted like this, but after the baby comes you'll probably look back on these early weeks as hugely peaceful. Right now you may feel pretty anxious, uncertain, disoriented. For peace of mind, reach out to your source of spiritual strength.

THOUGHT FOR TODAY: Clearing my life of unproductive worry is the most healing thing I can do for my baby and me.

Day 16

How did the stalks of rye know about bearing grain? And how did the wheat know about reproducing itself? No—they didn't know. They did it instinctively.

—ISAAC BASHEVIS SINGER

Instinct is a dangerous word. It's been used to keep women in second place for a long time: "They have a mothering instinct, instead of a business one." No one says that fathering is instinctive, yet certainly men are as ready to begin babies as women are to carry them. Our bodies go through their marvelous biological tricks whether we have a mothering instinct or not. Both you and your partner have the ability to be parents, just as you're able to grow hair, but that doesn't mean that growing hair—or even growing a new life—is the basic function in your lives.

Remember always that you are choosing to mother this new life. Your baby may be growing without conscious decisions on your part; you may even bond with your child without willing it. But this pregnancy is your choice. Other choices are yours as well, and will be your child's.

THOUGHT FOR TODAY: The world needs to take the right perspective on motherhood: it's a privilege, not a sentence.

> *Thou clarity,*
> *That with angelic charity*
> *Revealest beauty where thou art,*
> *Spread thyself like a clean pool.*
> —ANNA HEMPSTEAD BRANCH

Your life is the same, only different. Many women find the difference confusing at times. It's normal to long for clarity, for an answer to the confusion.

Part of what you're feeling may be chemical: your hormones have changed. The tiny sac surrounding your baby is secreting chorionic gonadotropin, the pregnancy hormone. It's this substance in your blood or urine that gives the diagnosis of pregnancy in the first place, and undoubtedly it has some effect on your body's usual hormonal mix.

Whether it's chemical or psychological, or a combination of both, your confusion is natural. Making a quiet space in your mind and spirit for a little time each day will help you sort out your thoughts and feelings, and when you achieve some clarity within yourself, you're better able to accept the uncontrollable future. What will happen, will happen.

THOUGHT FOR TODAY: I have the power to accept the changes that come to me, with each new mixture of hormones, and my baby will go on growing. We're both doing the best we can.

Day 18

The shortest way to do many things is to do only one thing at once.

—RICHARD CECIL

When I was a child I remember grown-ups telling me, "One thing at a time! Finish one thing before you start another!" Later, I read somewhere that you can't truly do two things at the same time; you may think you're watching TV while you read, but you're really reading and watching alternately—like patting your stomach and rubbing your head.

Right now you really *are* doing several things simultaneously—leading your ordinary life of work and leisure and relationships, while at the same time you are developing internally in new ways, nourishing your baby, and helping it grow a beautiful, complex little body.

But the grown-ups were right, of course; it's not really you that is doing all these things, but the power of life itself. These things happen to us and through us; the power ensures that your muscles and brain cells know what to do to accommodate your baby, and that it knows how to grow.

THOUGHT FOR TODAY: My baby's human program proceeds under a greater guidance than I could provide. I can relax into my life, knowing we're well looked after.

> *Expectation is a thin honey on our skin.*
> *It's something like the storm's approach*
> *a tense green violet*
> *over the stillness of the water's teal.*
> —LAURA CHESTER

I remember when I was a child, feeling anxious and crowded by adults' expectations of me. I knew I could always do better if no one was paying any particular attention. And my own expectations still mainly get in my way; impromptu parties are more fun than planned ones. Of course, impromptu parties work better when there's a good supply of food, drink, and interesting people.

In this pregnancy as in the rest of life, you'll do best if you let go of any particular expectations. Take good care of yourself, but don't fall into the trap of expecting perfection in return. Expectations set you up for disappointments. If you do your part with an open heart and a positive, loving attitude, you can't be disappointed.

THOUGHT FOR TODAY: I am strong and will do my best and whatever happens will be for the best. I'm responsible for the effort, not the outcome.

> *I am an instrument in the shape*
> *of a woman trying to translate pulsations*
> *into images for the relief of the body*
> *and the reconstruction of the mind*
> —ADRIENNE RICH

One woman said, "For hours at a time, I forget about my little clot, little freckle, and then I remember, with a thrill of secret pleasure. But sometimes my pleasure is tinged with worry, still. What if my test results are false-positives? What if something's wrong?"

In a few weeks, you'll be able to see an ultrasound scan of your baby, and that may give you a stronger sense of its reality. Some women are sure they can sense the baby, in the tenderness of their breasts, or in the leaden fatigue they feel every afternoon. Others say they feel as they always did, safe and single in their bodies. The dotted pattern on the ultrasound scan doesn't have any relation to a baby. It's still more an ideal project than a concrete reality.

At times it may be difficult to accept that all is well, and this pregnancy is going just as it should. Your doctor can put your mind at rest, and you can soothe your spirit.

THOUGHT FOR TODAY: Whatever uncertainty you're feeling, don't worry. It's right for you, right now.

Day 21

At the beginning of the nineteenth century, white American women bore an average of more than seven live children. . . . Pregnancy, birth, and postpartum recovery occupied a significant portion of most women's adult lives, and motherhood defined a major part of their identity.
—JUDITH WALZER LEAVITT

Pregnancy—the physical process—is the same for you as it was for your remotest ancestors. Medieval women, tribal women, hominid women all went through the same sequence of missed periods, weight gain, and the final unmistakable evidence of the baby moving within.

Tribal women may have had a safer time in childbirth than our eighteenth- and nineteeth-century "civilized" forebears, because they were probably attended by midwives or wisewomen, who knew much about cleanliness and medicinal herbs. Medicine in later centuries was pretty barbarous in comparison, and childbirth was dangerous. It's interesting to see that the cycle of wisdom is moving back in that direction, with nurse-midwives, birthing rooms, and the custom of having friends as well as spouses attend the birth.

The important difference is that you have choices—choice of how you'll give birth, and choice of whether to let motherhood define your identity for a few months or a lifetime. This choice represents the most striking change in women's lives in all history.

THOUGHT FOR TODAY: I'm grateful that I have choices, and I'll use them responsibly.

Day 22

> *Now almost everything I ever imagined*
> *Has caught up with me . . .*
> —PATRICIA GOEDICKE

In high school, some girls talked about pregnancy as "getting caught"—as though our experiments in sexual loving were a game of tag, with pregnancy as a penalty. You may feel caught, now, too, caught up in a silken net of necessity. The difference is that you've chosen to wear this net. You can take pride in your position; rather than losing, you've won something. This pregnancy is something that involves you in body, mind, heart, and spirit. You bring to it everything you have and everything you are.

The new life within you can indeed be almost everything you ever imagined. It may belong in part to your fantasies of sickness and weakness; but it can also belong to the realm of creation and fruitful possibility. All your fears, hopes, and desires are echoed in this process. Don't be afraid of feeling whatever you feel. It will take you a while to get used to the idea of your baby, and meanwhile your imagination is working overtime.

THOUGHT FOR TODAY: Nothing in our lives ever leaves us, unless we consciously choose to let it go. I'll exercise my powers of holding on and of releasing.

Day 23

> *Warmth   moisture*
> *Stir of incipient life*
> *Precipitating into me*
> *The contents of the universe*
> —MINA LOY

Sometime very soon, your baby's heart will form—little separate chambers, to pump blood that nourishes the brain, nerves, and muscles. Soon, in fact, its heartbeat will be audible. How will it feel to listen to this evidence, from deep inside your own body, of another heart beating?

This miracle is ordinary—as ordinary as a garden. Remember the incredible thrill of planting your first packet of seeds, and watching them grow? Mine were marigolds, my seventh summer. From watching them I came to understand that real miracles happen all the time.

The new life that started with the union of two single cells is already quite a miraculous being. As it grows, it will only become more so.

THOUGHT FOR TODAY: One of the gifts of pregnancy is making me pay attention to the many ordinary miracles present in my life.

Day 24

The tiny share we have of time appalls me, though my father who sometimes seems to have been at home as long as it has lasted, has really lived on this earth only a little longer than I have in terms of all the time there has been to live in.
—ALICE MUNRO

Do you remember the phrase from high-school biology, "Ontogeny recapitulates phylogeny"? It means that the stages of human growth echo or mirror the development of the human species, and your baby's growth has already followed this pattern. It has been more like a fish or a bird than a mammal, but by now it's already grown into an air-breathing, ovulating creature—one of us.

How many million years did it take for human beings to become what we are now? How many hundreds of thousands of years did our species spend stooped over, naked, eating leaves and grass? In a few thousand years we have whizzed from apelike creatures to voyagers in space.

We still have bodies and nervous systems that belong to simpler life-styles, and civilization can be hard on us. Praying and turning over our worries to a power greater than all of us, greater even than the differences between species, can keep us safe.

THOUGHT FOR TODAY: I will remember what makes us different from the animals, and how important it is to tend to our spiritual needs.

Day 25

Do I contradict myself? Very well then, I contradict myself. I am large, I contain multitudes.

—Walt Whitman

When you think of the next eight months and what is waiting for you at the end of them, do you have a vision of a perfect family: mom and dad and baby, neatly snuggled into a frame, bathed in golden light? Or do you feel as though you have been given a sentence at indentured labor?

Sometimes carrying your baby around may feel like punishment, at other times a rich reward. Perhaps you're going through mood changes, and seldom have the same feelings two days in a row. Many women report feeling out of control, swinging wildly between emotional extremes.

Peace and serenity may depend on accepting the fact that you are out of control, swept up in a vast and graceful project that is directed by forces greater than your individual self. Accepting the emotional changes of your pregnancy—whether they are perceived more as reward or punishment—depends largely on you. You can summon whatever response you desire, for you do contain multitudes.

THOUGHT FOR TODAY: I can't control my contradictory feelings, but I can control my response to them.

Day 26

The first law of ecology is that everything is related to everything else.

—BARRY COMMONER

Through this pregnancy you can discover new connections with parts of the world that may have seemed very distant from you before—a new awareness is being born.

When you read about hunger in Asia or India—or even, shamefully, in your own country—you now know what it means for a poor woman to try to feed her children. You know too that if a woman who doesn't get enough to eat becomes pregnant, the growing child within her will suffer.

You may even look at eggs differently, and at chickens and all the other animal foods we eat. They're connected to the cycle of birth and growth. Quarts of milk wouldn't be on the supermarket shelves if cows didn't have hormones very like the ones that are readying your breasts to give milk.

Women are thought to have been the first gardeners in prehistoric times. It's probably because our bodies contain some knowledge about growing things and feeding people.

THOUGHT FOR TODAY: I'm happy to feel more closely related to other cycles of birth and growth.

Day 27

I'll walk where my own nature would be leading,
It vexes me to choose another guide:
Where the gray flocks in ferny glens are feeding;
Where the wild wind blows on the mountain side.
                                            —EMILY BRONTË

"Eat this, read that, have you bought thus-and-so?" We are bombarded on all sides with advertisements and advice, so much so that sometimes we forget where our own natures would be leading us. We need to go deep within ourselves, to tap our own connection to a source of spiritual strength, in order to reassure ourselves that all the help we want or need is close at hand, close as your heartbeat, close as my breath.

Your baby is a tiny fishlike creature growing inside you, changing more rapidly than a tadpole or minnow, spinning through thousands of years of human evolution in these short weeks. You are becoming its mother, a role you've never played before. Your best guide is your trusted inner voice. Your own nature tells you to rely on the nourishment that has sustained you in the past—not ignoring well-meant advice, but supplementing it with what you already know.

THOUGHT FOR TODAY: My physical and spiritual health depends on my balancing my internal sense of rightness with trusted advice from outside. I pray for the wisdom to do this.

Mbuti see their life as beginning the moment they were wanted, for that is when they were conceived, and from these stories told them throughout childhood all Mbuti have a detailed, though not necessarily exact or verifiable, knowledge of their earliest beginnings.

—COLIN TURNBULL

This is an interesting pun on the word *preconceptions*. You conceived of your baby long before it was actually conceived. Maybe its life did begin as soon as you thought of it; in one sense, you taught yourself to want a baby from your thoughts and dreams, and your notions of what your child is will shape it as certainly as the nucleic acids in your chromosomes.

You and your partner will tell your baby stories of its earliest beginnings, of how you wanted it and talked about it even before you brought it into being. Your child will learn who she or he is at least partly from hearing about who you are.

Children love to hear stories about their origins; from such stories and dreams of desire they learn that you can have whatever you deeply want, with both your body and your spirit.

THOUGHT FOR TODAY: I will be sure that my preconceived notions and desires don't interfere with my seeing who my child really is.

Day 29

Mothering invites the habit of prayer for prayer is a natural builder of self-confidence. . . . Prayer is a great relaxation technique.

—MURSHIDA VERA JUSTIN CORDA

A year ago you weren't pregnant, yet you still needed to plan relaxation in your life. A month ago you weren't pregnant, yet you may have prayed. The simplest prayer can put you in touch with your source of love and creativity, the calm deep well that you can always tap when you need refreshment.

These months of pregnancy can be a time of spiritual growth and renewal. Use them to strengthen your connections. Half an hour—even fifteen minutes—of quiet reflection can refresh your spirit and your body, too.

In preparation for labor and delivery, you'll be learning relaxation techniques to help you surrender to the birth process and cooperate with it. Your muscles can learn to accommodate your new state, and you can participate best through prayer and meditation.

THOUGHT FOR TODAY: When I am deep in prayer I am not only soothing my spirit, I am also aiding my physical adjustment to this pregnancy.

> *. . . I am faithful to*
> *ebb and flow, I fall*
> *in season and now*
>
> *is a time of ripening.*
> —DENISE LEVERTOV

The first missed period is the sign most women wait for—yet perhaps you don't fully trust it. The language of the body is sometimes clear but sometimes cryptic. Your hormonal cycle is delicate, and it may respond to many things in your life—work stress, emotional pressure, happiness, travel, the flu—in ways you can't always understand.

Your body is faithful to ebb and flow, and instead of shedding your extra richness, your body is using it to nourish your baby. Your baby is ripening like a little fruit or a nut inside the safe shell of your abdominal wall. You shelter it with your flesh and bones but also with your heart, brain, and spirit.

You are ripening together in this phase of your growth cycle. Silently your baby connects you to yourself, to others, and to the future; without your conscious knowledge you help it to build itself.

THOUGHT FOR TODAY: Like a ripe fruit, my baby will fall in season, a time of joyful harvest.

Day 31

The peace of great changes be for you.
Whisper, Oh beginners in the hills.
Tumble, Oh cubs—tomorrow belongs to you.
— CARL SANDBURG

Great changes bring peace to a well-nourished spirit, because it surrenders to them. The rhythm of great change has already begun for you, letting you know in subtle ways that you are taking your place in the pattern of generations.

Tomorrow may belong to your baby's contemporaries, but today is yours, and today you can begin the spiritual surrender that brings peace. The past is past; the future will unfold in time; but the present moment is yours. You have the choice of cluttering your life with worries or regrets, or turning them over to the care of a power greater than yourself.

You'll have many decisions to make in the course of your pregnancy—choice of birth advisors, where to give birth, whether to breast-feed your baby, whether to allow the many advanced techniques for monitoring the course of your pregnancy, labor, and delivery, as well as the day-to-day decisions about food, clothes, work, and leisure that are affected by your newest great change. It's up to you whether you make them peacefully, based on your knowledge and feelings, or let yourself feel overwhelmed by them.

THOUGHT FOR TODAY: I can accept great changes in peace, because I trust in my higher power to guide my decisions.

THIS MONTH'S VISIT TO THE DOCTOR

Date:

Weight: Blood Pressure:

Weight Gain:

This Month's Signs of Pregnancy:

Changes in Eating:

Changes in Sleeping:

Changes in Activities/Energy Level:

Reflections:

Questions for Next Month's Visit:

Day 1

Why are we
Already mother-creatures, double-bearing,
With matrices in body and in brain?
—AMY LOWELL

In Latin *matrix* means womb; in printing, it means the mat or ground that receives impressions; in mathematics, it's the field in which operations take place. The human brain seems to have a readiness for learning language that could be called a matrix.

Your body has always had this matrix, this capacity for mothering, this power to generate a new life, just as your brain has always been able to grasp the concept of motherhood. Until now, this was a readiness; now, it's an actuality.

There's nothing passive about your readiness, although your baby's growth is happening without your conscious participation. Your conscious behavior is vital to your welfare and to your baby's. You're a team, a unit. How well you do depends a lot on how smoothly you partner each other. You need to listen closely to your body; pay attention to the skilled advice of your childbirth advisors, whether they are obstetrician-gynecologists, nurse-midwives, or alternative healers; and call, when you need to, on your source of spiritual strength.

THOUGHT FOR TODAY: My capacity for mothering can bring me both pleasure and power. I will practice partnering with my baby now.

Day 2

I remember greeting the certitude of the belated child's presence with serious mistrust, while saying nothing about it. Physical apprehension had nothing to do with my behavior; I was simply afraid that at my age I would not know how to give a child the proper love and care, devotion and understanding.
—COLETTE

For many women, this is a serious worry. Some say it's almost their first response to the thought that they might be pregnant. Almost. First there is a slash of pure joy or pure terror, then the worry: me? How can I do this? I don't know how.

When you take some deep, calming breaths and set your worry on one side, you might remind yourself that no one knows before the fact; no one is ever ready to give a baby what it deserves. A child deserves everything: peace, abundance, infinite love, and care. This child of yours will be born into an imperfect world, with parents who are imperfect people. You may not have the knowledge, the patience, the boundless devotion your baby deserves. Remember, you are just the best mother it will have, and you're doing the best you can.

If you can reach a deeper level of tranquillity and open yourself to the possibilities of motherhood, you'll probably acknowledge that your best is good enough, as your mother's best was, in the end, good enough for you.

THOUGHT FOR TODAY: I am here, alive and well and carrying a new life. I will know what I need to know.

Day 3

Babies should grow in fields;
common as beets or turnips
they should be picked and held
root end up, soil spilling
from between their toes—
                            —LINDA PASTAN

Will your baby be round and rosy, gurgling to itself and happy as a puppy or a kitten? Or will it be a pale, slow baby, or a delicate baby, quick to startle or to cry? Of course, you're curious about your baby; you are going to be together for the next umpteen years.

All the books say you'll "bond," whatever that is—sounds like epoxy resin in a tube—so you probably don't have to worry about loving your baby enough. But many expectant mothers worry that their babies will pick up on all the things about themselves that they don't like. Fussy eating, impatience, sloppiness, whatever a woman dislikes in herself or her partner, she fears to find again in the new baby.

It's well to remember that worrying about what you can't control is simply a way of making yourself unhappy. During this pregnancy you can choose to be happy.

THOUGHT FOR TODAY: Life has been matching mothers and babies for a long, long time. Why shouldn't I expect success?

Day 4

Every woman has a history
mother and grandmother and the ones before that
the faces she sees in dreams or visions
and wonders Who?

—SHARON BARBA

Your baby's eyes are forming. The delicate neural mechanism that receives images of the world is taking shape these days, although the information for interpreting these images will develop much later. Human eyes are constructed something like cameras, with lenses and "light meters"—the way our pupils dilate or contract. No one knows whether your baby "sees" anything inside you, or whether its brain can form images before it has any experience of the world.

Perhaps we'll never understand just what are the contents of a newborn human's mind—where is the line between an instinct and an idea, for example; and how can it recognize your smell and the taste of your milk? Does its brain already contain the image of a human face, so it will know you when it sees you?

Everything that happens to your baby is part of its history, even now, even today, when it isn't much bigger than your eye. The food you eat and the air you breathe nourish it. Why not decide that everything you see is communicated to your baby?

THOUGHT FOR TODAY: My baby and I deserve the best: excellent nourishment, and harmony and loveliness in what we see.

Day 5

*There are only two sorts of doctors: those who practice with
their brains, and those who practice with their tongues.*
                                                —Sir William Osler

Now is the time for you to decide on your source of
prenatal care. You need a health advisor who practices with
both brain and tongue. One healer might be brilliant, but if
she or he doesn't communicate, you won't get the full benefit
of that brilliance.

The most important thing is for you to feel comfortable
with your care provider. You've probably heard all sorts of
stories from your friends and family: the obstetrician who calls
his patients "my girls" and makes up their minds for them
about whether they need painkillers; the nurse-midwife who
after delivery always looks damp, radiant, and gloriously
disheveled, as though she'd given birth herself. There's a
whole movement devoted to birthing in water, an idea that
strikes some women as marvelous and some as loony. Be
assured that fashions in health care may come and go, but
ultimately you'll decide what's best for you. If you need help
in making a decision, many resources are constantly available
to you.

THOUGHT FOR TODAY: I will look for the balance of
authority and independence that most empowers me to give
birth as I wish.

Day 6

> *All things move toward*
> *the light*
>
> *except those*
> *that freely work down*
>
> *to oceans' black depths*
> —LORINE NIEDECKER

Before your baby can move toward the light, it must stay in the secure nest you provide. Right now, it is a creature of darkness and might as well be at the bottom of the ocean, but the effect this pregnancy is having on your life can fill it with light—the light of expanded consciousness, as well as joy.

Beyond the details, morning nausea and hospital insurance, where to put the cradle, how long to breast-feed, the new life sheds a radiance into your life. Birth is one of the sacred events, and these days you are living close to holiness. You may not consciously feel it all the time, but you deserve to cherish it.

Above all, make sure that in your joyful concentration on the new life, you never lose sight of yourself, your own ongoing life and relationships. In the moments you set aside for spiritual renewal, allow yourself to feel the radiance. It will transform you.

THOUGHT FOR TODAY: I deserve to enjoy everything that happens in this process, for I've been touched by holiness.

Day 7

"If I'd stayed home to take care of a child I'd have ended up hating him, and he'd have had to grow up with that, too. Like a lot of these kids who had their mother's devotion and her secret hatred."

—Vivian Gornick

Many women don't have the luxury of choosing whether or not to stay home with a new baby; either they must return to work as soon as they can or they are expected to stay in the home. In neither case does the woman decide freely that this is the best decision for herself and her child.

All mothers and babies are alike in the big ways—our pregnancies follow the same course, and our lactation; there are only so many ways to labor and give birth—but we're all different, too. Different patterns of work inside and outside of the home correspond with these differences. Every woman has individual needs, and all families develop their own patterns for fulfillment. You and your partner will find the balance that's right for the two of you and your child.

Whatever your decision, your inner guide will let you know if it's the right one. When you make the choice that best meets your needs for combining work and love, you'll feel peaceful and harmonious. Of course, there will be anxieties and conflicts; they're a part of life.

THOUGHT FOR TODAY: I feel lucky to have the choices I have, and I trust that my overall sense will guide me.

Day 8

Very few things happen at the right time, and the rest do not happen at all.

—HERODOTUS

Did you and your partner intend to get pregnant right now, at this exact moment? What about everything else in your lives—other children, jobs, travel, money, parents' health?

No matter how carefully you may have planned this, it's normal to have some doubts about your timing. But apparently the time was right for your baby and for the forces that combined to start a new life, and if you will accept that, it becomes right for you, as well.

You have the power to decide that your pregnancy happened at the right time. Only if you want to punish yourself will you struggle against acceptance of your new family life. You deserve to have peace and joy with this pregnancy, and positive acceptance will help you toward this goal.

THOUGHT FOR TODAY: Perhaps, if I had not conceived when I did, I might not have conceived at all. Here, as in other areas of my life, I willingly surrender control to the power that is wiser than I.

Day 9

They say that there are no such wild speculators as women. It seems easy to them that a sort of miracle should happen; that something should come out of nothing.

—MARGARET OLIPHANT

Your baby didn't come out of nothing, and it's not growing without help. Its body is growing on the same nourishment your body uses to keep itself going; that's why it is so important for you to eat well, whole grains and beans, fresh fruits and vegetables, pure meat and fish, cheese, yogurt, milk, eggs from healthy chickens. Meals should be simple, carefully prepared to give you what you need. Women used to say, "A tooth is lost for every child," because when they didn't get enough calcium in their diets, the growing baby's bones and teeth depleted the mother's own calcium reserves.

It's still a miracle, how neatly and precisely your cells perform their programmed work. Your baby's brain, heart, and digestive system are already forming, and its endocrine glands have begun to develop. The chorionic sac is already doing its valuable work of bringing oxygen and nutrients to your baby from your bloodstream and carrying carbon dioxide and other metabolic wastes back to you—because you can get rid of them, by breathing out and excreting. Miraculous!

THOUGHT FOR TODAY: Since the human species can do these wonders, perhaps we can do even more. The world needs more peace and love—I'll direct my thoughts toward these miracles, too.

Day 10

Whoever could make two ears of corn, or two blades of grass, to grow upon a spot of ground where only one grew before, would . . . do more essential service . . . than the whole race of politicians put together.

—JONATHAN SWIFT

The sacred texts of most faiths include some directions about maintaining the population of the faithful; for example, the god of the Old Testament instructed his people to increase and multiply. Which is exactly what you're doing—essential service to the human race. You deserve to feel absolutely right within yourself, dutiful and good.

Yours is good work, the best there is, and as a vital worker you deserve the best—the best care, the best nurture, the best growing conditions for your precious project. Your loved ones do their best, but it's really up to you to safeguard the quality of your life. You can start by working on your attitude: the highest quality of experience isn't attained by accident. To receive love, you must be loving; to position yourself for grace, you must be gracious.

THOUGHT FOR TODAY: I'm bearing this child for my family and my society, but most of all for myself, and we deserve the highest quality of life. Excellence comes from choices I make.

Day 11

Tranquil well of deep delight,
Transparent as the water, bright—
All things that shine through thee appear
As stones through water, sweetly clear.
—ANNA HEMPSTEAD BRANCH

Everyone has down days, and they don't go away just because you're pregnant. Even without morning sickness or fatigue, there are some days when every mistake you ever made comes back to haunt you. It may seem impossible that you will give birth to a baby who will grow up to be a good human being . . . or even that you will survive your child's infancy without going mad.

On the bleakest days, remember that your baby is growing as it needs to grow, taking the best ingredients it can from what's offered. Your child is programmed for excellence; its life before birth will have accustomed it to the best.

You could try to start each day with consciousness of your child, reminding yourself that any sickness or wooziness you feel is evidence that it's taking care of itself. You're part of this process, but you can't control it completely.

THOUGHT FOR TODAY: Whatever doubts I may have about this pregnancy, I can resolve them by remembering that my baby is already preparing itself for health and well-being.

Day 12

Today when I see "truthful"
written somewhere, it flares

like a white orchid in wet woods,
*   rare and grief-delighting, up from the page.*
Sometimes, unwittingly even,
*   we have been truthful.*
In a random universe, what more

exact and starry consolation?
                                        —ADRIENNE RICH

Truth begins with the self. For you to be truthful means admitting the whole bewildering mixture of what you feel: delight, anxiety, anger sometimes, love, fear, irritation, great happiness. No one else can speak exactly to your condition, nor can you speak to anyone else's.

Fortunately, you share a language with millions of other people that lets us communicate some small part of our truth. If you speak carefully, you can achieve truth in your speech. But communication between you and your baby, because it is utterly wordless, is always and only the truth.

Words can never be as exact as your wordless communication, but you can still resolve to be truthful always with your child. This is the highest form of respect you can give to another person. You'll ask no less from your child.

THOUGHT FOR TODAY: My baby will never learn falsehood from me. Together we'll learn to speak the truth.

Day 13

Good and evil, dead and alive, everything blooms
From one natural stem.

—RUMI

The little stalk that grows into your baby's placenta is that natural stem. Everything in the world bloomed from it. No wonder pregnant women were worshipped in ancient times.

One can understand how men might envy women's ability to nurture new life. If the men in your life seem preoccupied or angry sometimes, maybe—on some level they're not even conscious of—they're feeling something like that envy. Or maybe they're fully aware of it, experiencing jealousy, wondering what it feels like to be pregnant, wishing they could do it, too.

This is the one power women have that men can never have—bearing children, nursing them from our bodies. Your understanding can bring you closer to the men you love, instead of driving you apart. After your child is born, its father can be as close to it as he wants; in some families, fathers even become the primary care givers. But he and the baby will never be two blossoms on one stem, as you and it are now.

THOUGHT FOR TODAY: After the birth, this relation will change along with everything else. Let me wear this power lightly, for it is my strength.

Day 14

You and your baby will have been together for a long time before you ever touch hands. Your baby's hands—those marvelous human instruments—are forming this month, though its fingers and toes are still webbed, like a little amphibian's. You can't touch it with your hands until it is born, but you touch it now in intimate, vital ways, through your heart's blood, your brain waves, your breath, your pulse.

When you were a baby, doctors believed that few substances passed from mother to baby, but now we know that there is no barrier between us. Future investigators may find that some diseases and allergies come from some combination of infants' genetic predisposition and mothers' behavior during pregnancy.

These months together will stamp your baby as a member of your family, no matter what it looks like. Everything you do now is probably communicated to your baby, including many things that seem to have little meaning—your body's movements when you walk or dance, your choice of flavorings in food, perhaps even the books you read or films you see.

THOUGHT FOR TODAY: I hope that the foods, music, and thoughts I can enjoy will affect my baby positively. I'll devote my days to finding suitable, compatible nourishment.

Day 15

Spirit children who are great friends and always in pairs are choosy about being born again; life with their friends in the spirit world is comfortable and moreover there is the danger of losing one's twin-friend during the journey, since it is rare for a spirit-pair to agree to enter a single womb.

—ROBERT BRAIN

This story about how twins come to be is charming, although the actual prospect of having twins may be terrifying. It is a sweet idea to think of souls being twinned; one of the quests in one's life after birth might be to find one's twin-friend.

Twin births are fairly rare, only about one in one hundred and eighty births for U.S. mothers. If your family has twins in it, or your partner's family does, that shortens your odds. There are plenty of stories about women who didn't know they were carrying twins until delivery, but in most twin pregnancies both heartbeats can be clearly heard and an ultrasound scan usually is definitive.

If yours is a twin pregnancy, you will probably know it very soon. And you'll have seven months or so to get used to the idea. You will need all your powers of relaxation and surrender to help you bear and nurture twin babies, but you will be equal to whatever comes.

THOUGHT FOR TODAY: My faith in the goodness of life can sustain me through tasks that would seem infinitely complicated and difficult without it.

Day 16

> *Women sit in the balance, as*
> *Upon a knife;*
> *Irony cuts to the quick—is this*
> *Life or new life?*
> —BARBARA HOWES

For some women, pregnancy is a frightening possibility. Every menstrual period is greeted with relief by a woman who lacks the resources, internal or external, to rear children properly. You are fortunate indeed to be able to rejoice in the new life.

The world's abundance could give all women joy in their fertility, but our wealth is badly distributed, and many have none. During the next months, whatever happens remember your good fortune. And if you choose to put your energy into bringing about more just and equitable arrangements for mothers and babies, however you can, you'll be amply repaid. All new lives deserve to be safeguarded as lovingly as yours.

THOUGHT FOR TODAY: In my own happiness, I won't forget the many mothers who must see their children hungry and sick, and the many more women who fear the very blessing I rejoice in.

Day 17

And when the great moment came and went in a fairly regular fashion, the neighbors recognized that for all their expectations a baby was a baby.

—BONNIE G. SMITH

Many pregnant women feel a lot of pressure from the grandparents-to-be, who sometimes act as though no one ever had a baby before. It's probably better for them to make a fuss over you than to ignore you, although you may definitely feel harassed when mother and mother-in-law call every week to hear what you're eating, how you're sleeping, whether you throw up in the mornings, and what kinds of vitamins you're taking.

In old stories about prophecies, we read that people have sometimes decided newborn babies were going to be kings or murderers, criminals or saviors. Your baby has the capacity to be any of those things (well, maybe not a king). Every child that's born is entitled to the best the world can offer.

Your child will be born at a time of shrinking population in some parts of the world, exploding population in others. While your child will be precious to you, to the world it will be another mouth to feed, another bottom to diaper, another consumer of goods and generator of garbage. One of your tasks as a mother will be to raise a thoughtful, caring world citizen—part of the solution to the world's woes, not another problem.

THOUGHT FOR TODAY: My child will learn about responsibility from me, as well as privilege.

Day 18

It's all a world where bugs and emperors
Go singularly back to the same dust,
Each in his time.
— EDWIN ARLINGTON ROBINSON

We are headed for a time when more human beings are alive on the planet at once than have ever lived before. You can't give mental space or energy to all those others who breathe the same air, and drink the same water, but for your baby's sake, you'd better make the effort to think a bit about how your individual decisions affect the world we share.

Every time you throw away a piece of plastic, you're adding to the chlorofluorocarbons that are released when they're incinerated; these CFCs weaken our atmosphere's protective ozone layer. This kind of thinking should be a factor in such decisions as whether to buy disposable diapers for your baby or use a diaper service or launder your own cloth diapers.

Your baby will be born into a very different world from the world of your infancy. Our society is aging, as more older people live longer, but in other societies children make up a greater share of the population. We own much of the world's wealth and it's our responsibility to use our prosperity responsibly.

THOUGHT FOR TODAY: My baby will help me make decisions that are healthy for our world, as well as for its precious self.

Day 19

You must know your own need,
You must nakedly dare
To form a perfect deed,
To fruit a spirit fair.
— Elizabeth Daryush

It's tempting to fantasize about your baby's future—how good-looking, intelligent, successful it will be, how proud and happy it will make you. These daydreams aren't prophecies; they are thinly disguised wishes, and they express more about you than about your baby.

The best work you can do now for your child's future is to attend to your own well-being, to address your spiritual hungers and find ways of satisfying them. Knowing your own needs for love and admiration, your desire for recognition, you can go where you will find it—to those who love and admire you, those family members and friends who value you. And you can also learn to love and admire yourself.

This last is key, for if you lack a good opinion of yourself, you're not likely to believe anything anyone tells you; your deepest hunger will go unappeased, and you may try to find vicarious satisfaction through your child. Satisfying your own need for love will give you the grace and strength to satisfy your child's.

THOUGHT FOR TODAY: I must be wonderful; I'm my baby's mother.

Day 20

*Now that I had learned that women and children carried the
heaviest burden of our ruthless economic system, I saw that it
was a mockery to expect them to wait until the social
revolution arrives in order to right injustice.*

—EMMA GOLDMAN

Our market economy can be ruthless, and the poor, by
and large, are women and their children. Even as you rejoice
over your baby and the life to come, you know that too many
women who are pregnant like you are too young or too poor,
or both, to give their babies the quality of life you want for
your child.

You want to have the best prenatal care, the safest and
most accurate kind of monitoring before and during the birth.
After your child is born it deserves the gentlest, wisest care in
health and sickness: prompt immunizations, the best nutrition, the most loving and intelligent training, whether it is
provided by you or someone else. All mothers want the same
things for their babies, but most can't afford them.

The United States has shockingly high infant mortality for
the world's richest country, most of it due to lack of prenatal
care for young and poor mothers. Things need to change, so
more people can share in our good luck. Whether or not you
believe we need a "social revolution," you know that mothers
and babies deserve the best.

THOUGHT FOR TODAY: I will support improvements in
health and welfare, and candidates who believe as I do, to
help bring about a world where all mothers and children get
what they need.

Day 21

"What's miraculous about a spider's web," said Mrs. A-rable. "I don't see why you say a web is a miracle—it's just a web."
"Ever try to spin one?"

—E. B. WHITE

Many pregnant women say that even though they may still feel sickish in the mornings and sometimes dizzy and exhausted in the afternoons, even though they fall asleep reading, watching television, or in the middle of a conversation, even though they can't quite succeed in feeling beautiful, this is a very happy time. They have the consciousness of a wonderful secret inside of them, miraculous as a mother spider's delicate web.

Your baby is still just an embryo; it hasn't been promoted yet to a fetus. It doesn't even have a placenta, just a membranous sac called the chorionic vesicle, filled with fluids that bathe its tiny body. Your baby is connected to this sac by a body stalk, like a little sweet pea; later, the stalk will develop into its umbilical cord.

You probably read some of these words and images in high school or college biology courses. They may have seemed boring or disgusting at the time; now they seem beautiful.

THOUGHT FOR TODAY: I have shared my secret with the people I love most, but I know they probably don't really understand the silent, miraculous spinning of our web.

Day 22

Every being cries out to be read differently.
                              —Simone Weil

There's nothing much that's new about pregnancy. Any doctor you consult will have seen it all before; your parents went through it; probably many of your friends have had the experience. You can't reasonably expect anybody but your immediate family to share your excitement. Yet this *is* different, because it's yours, and you've never done this before. This pregnancy must be read differently from all those millions of others, although in many ways it is the same.

Being pregnant gives you kinship with every woman who ever has been pregnant. You understand what it feels like to miss your menstrual periods and to have a new life growing inside you. At the same time, you know everything in your life is different and unique, because it's yours; it's never happened quite this way before.

THOUGHT FOR TODAY: My hope is that mine will be a healthy baby, just like millions of others, and unlike anyone who ever lived.

Day 23

It is not at all uncommon for a man to go through a pregnancy with his wife in a quite literal fashion . . . essentially a "birth-giving gesture" on the part of the father who found mere procreation emotionally insufficient, and who sought to share the birth experience to bind himself more closely to his child.

—NANCY CALDWELL SOREL

In some cultures, this gesture is recognized in ceremonies and rituals called *couvade*, but in ours, men are left to work out their needs for sharing the experience pretty much on their own. Keep this phenomenon in mind; your partner may have a series of minor illnesses; he may gain or lose weight; if he's had back trouble in the past, it may flare up again.

These signs are all healthy, and they may all be expressions of his very real desires to share in your physical changes. (Of course, they're also illnesses or injuries that have to be dealt with in and of themselves.) In a very real sense, you are a pregnant couple.

The stronger his physical identification with your pregnancy, the more closely he's going to want to be involved with the baby's care. If you're ever tempted to tease or nag him for his couvade symptoms, remember to rejoice also in his eagerness to father the baby and to feed, bathe, diaper, and rock it.

THOUGHT FOR TODAY: Nothing that happens to either of us during pregnancy is trivial; we can use the opportunity to deepen our sympathy with one another.

Day 24

Never would my child wait outside my door for me to finish a nap, a phone conversation, a card game. I would undo, I would redo my childhood. I would do for my child what had never been done for me.

—ANNE ROIPHE

However wonderful our childhoods might have been, everyone feels their parents' work can be improved. A new baby gives us a chance to learn from their mistakes, we believe, a chance to give a child the total love and acceptance we didn't have.

Yet the only real training we get for raising our children is how we were raised ourselves; all new parents catch themselves in this paradox. Many couples have their bitterest fights about how to raise their children, so if you and your partner have different ideas, you should start working on compromises now.

Did your parents feel this way? No doubt—and, if some of the things they did with you were a reaction against things your grandparents did with them, perhaps you will find yourself agreeing with your grandparents. Then will your child react against that, as your parents did, and raise her or his children the way you were raised? This dynamic might explain why styles in child rearing change in cycles, from strict to permissive to disciplined to relaxed.

THOUGHT FOR TODAY: I'll pray not for perfection but for understanding and wisdom.

> *I am knowing*
> *All about*
> *   Unfolding*
> —Mina Loy

There is a system of movement called Continuum, in which the head, trunk, arms, and legs are moved very gently, with close attention to the space in which you are moving. Concentrating on slow and gradual movement opens up the sense of more space than we ordinarily imagine. Something as simple as turning your head can become a journey of discovery, if you do it with infinite slowness and smoothness, over about two minutes. Space unfolds; you feel like an explorer.

These exercises are especially good for pregnant women, because the imagination gets a workout as much as the body. See if you can find Continuum classes in your community. It will never replace more vigorous exercise, but it's a valuable supplement. Movement can put you in touch with other kinds of unfolding—the subtle opening and softening of your emotions, the tiny changes that are preparing you over these long months for your baby's birth.

THOUGHT FOR TODAY: When I raise my arm with infinite slowness, I think of my baby and its growth, so subtle that my senses can't perceive it. But my imagination can help me experience the change.

Day 26

"My God, the human baby! A few weeks after birth, any other animal can fend for itself. But you! A basket case till you're twenty-one!"

—MEGAN TERRY

Human babies take a long time to develop and grow, compared to other animals, because people are such splendidly complex creatures. We want our babies to be all they can be, however long it takes. Parents need patience and humility to remember this after their children are born.

In earlier centuries, people were expected to mature much more quickly. Often they married in their early teens and were parents several times over by the time they were twenty. Of course, life expectancy for most people was only about half of what your baby's will be. Styles of childhood and adolescence are culturally determined, not necessarily part of the human program.

Serene reflection will help you to accept the pace of your own growth, and your baby's, whatever it is. Stages of growth don't always come when we think we're ready for them. Sometimes they take us by surprise; often they feel long overdue.

THOUGHT FOR TODAY: I accept that the timing of our lives is not controlled by human wishes, and I work toward surrendering my desire for control.

> *I am an acme of things accomplished,*
> *and I am an encloser of things to be.*
> —WALT WHITMAN

Every day you have the right to say to yourself, "Well, you did good work today." The best work goes on not at your desk but inside you. The building of your baby's body, bones and brain and liver, is the best and most important work you have ever done. No wonder when a man wants to praise achievement as Whitman did, he borrows images of pregnancy. Tall buildings, complex machinery, great art, all seem insignificant compared to the incredible delicacy of your baby's body.

Every day you and your baby hit a new peak of your development, and you have a right to feel proud of every moment. My mother had a funny old friend who maintained that human beings reach their peak at the age of two; "It's all downhill from there," he'd say, shaking his head. You have a long way to go before you hit that one, and meanwhile each day is richer and fuller than the one before.

THOUGHT FOR TODAY: I can rejoice in our accomplishments so far while looking forward to even greater things ahead.

Day 28

A curious light has come over Dana these days, as if her pregnancy wasn't something she carried with her daily, but a new idea crossing her mind fresh and different each time. She often misses what I've said in conversation, her cues in the music when she's supposed to sing.

—Sara Vogan

For hours at a stretch you may not be aware of your baby's presence. When you get caught up in work or a book, a TV program or an intricate recipe, your mind isn't a pregnant mind. It's just the useful instrument it's always been for processing information and answering problems.

Then you remember, with a little shock of pleasure— something like a colored dye flooding a vat of water, purling into corners, making everything brighter. Your baby is there, though you can't see or feel it; your little companion soul, attached to you on the inside, making space in you where no space was before. The thought of it makes a similar space inside your mind, creating consciousness where before there was none.

These are twin miracles, one happening in your body and one in your spirit. Whether you pay attention to your baby all the time or not, it's there, deepening you.

THOUGHT FOR TODAY: Any time I want, I can dip down and touch my baby inside my mind, like a talisman.

Day 29

You day-sun, circling around,
You daylight, circling around,
You night-sun, circling around,
You poor body, circling around,
You wrinkled age, circling around,
You spotted with gray, circling around,
You wrinkled skin, circling around.
                    —SEMINOLE SONG

What goes around, comes around, they say. Everything we put into circulation returns to us, even new babies, for the world is a self-renewing system where the same elements recombine, decay, and form new combinations, endlessly we hope. Our flesh is built from the same elemental substances as earth and air; light and water nourish us all. We are brothers and sisters to one another and to the animals, birds, insects, and plants that share our atmosphere.

Each of us circles around, and within us circulate the words, feelings, impressions, and responses from which our culture is made. We create it, and we are created by it, in a never-ending reciprocity. Nothing is made from nothing, yet new combinations are constantly possible, constantly fresh. Each new arrangement of elements is unique, a cause for rejoicing.

THOUGHT FOR TODAY: When my baby is born, it will take its place in the circle, drawing from and adding to the continuity of our people.

Day 30

It is a noble thing, the rearing of warriors for the revolution. . . . You prepare yourself by being healthy and confident, by having options that give you confidence, by getting yourself together . . .

—TONI CADE BAMBARA

Your baby is a child of your fighting self as well as your loving self. It will be born from your flesh and spirit, and so you will bring forth a child from all of you—your doubts and self-mockery as well as your devotion and praise.

You can best prepare for your baby's coming by looking at your faith and your doubts. Where are you strong, how are you fearful? Can you support others in their struggles for independence, or must you struggle against them for control? Your baby will need to know how to stand as well as how to surrender, and you will want to share with it how you have surrendered and how you have stood fast.

Conflict is a part of life; blood is spilled at birth as well as at death. The rhythms of life destroy to create, then die to be born again. The most precious gift you can pass on to your baby is willingness to enter the stream of life, with its pain and delight. You can nourish your bodies with yogurt, whole grains, fruits, and leafy vegetables, and your spirit with reflection on the depth and richness of the choices that lie before you.

THOUGHT FOR TODAY: Your baby will be a warrior as well as a bringer of peace, for every creature struggles to survive. Birth will be the first victory.

Day 31

. . . through loving each other as we did, we offered a mirror, one to the other, through which to see ourselves in whole new ways.

—CAROL LEMIEUX

Having a baby never saved a marriage, and it never ruined one; but having a baby does permanently change all your relationships. You and your partner are already starting to see one another in whole new ways—as parents, as well as lovers, spouses, life partners.

Pregnancy and birth inevitably will strain your adjustment—your household routine as well as your emotional relationship. You may need to work out brand-new schedules for sharing work. Humor, patience, and faith in the genuineness of your love will sustain you.

Small conflicts can loom large in pregnancy, so the practice of detachment becomes important. You will need to practice clearing your mind of details and concentrating on reaching your place of calm. You will need to provide extra love and support.

Sharing the experience of pregnancy and birth will bring you and your partner closer together, if you both allow yourselves patience and humility. Loving relationships keep changing as long as they're alive. You can't control the changes, but you can enter them with your whole heart.

THOUGHT FOR TODAY: My baby's parents deserve the highest quality relationship, and my partner and I are working on it.

THIS MONTH'S VISIT TO THE DOCTOR

Date:

Weight: Blood Pressure:

Weight Gain:

This Month's Signs of Pregnancy:

Changes in Eating:

Changes in Sleeping:

Changes in Activities/Energy Level:

Reflections:

Questions for Next Month's Visit:

Day 1

Holding onto the fact
of her new life   is slippery   as the wet rail fence
she'd cross   going off
along through fields   away from it all
                                    —Laura Chester

At this stage of pregnancy many women, though they know they are pregnant, feel only the most slippery connection to their babies. You may know you're going to welcome it and mother it; you'll take joy in the birth and give your baby love and health. But at times you may feel the sadness that many pregnant women do, like a bass note under a melody, that underlies ordinary happiness.

This melancholy may stem partly from anxiety—you worry that you may not be the wonderful mother you want to be. And partly it may be anxiety for your baby, growing into the unknown. Partly, too, you may be grieving a little bit for the loss of your old life. However much you want the new life, some grief always accompanies profound change.

If you can, clear your mind of anxieties and try to touch the pure wonder of the new life inside yours. Imagine the stream of nourishment that flows from you to your baby as a clear river. More than blood filters across your membranes and into your baby's body; you transmit your thoughts and feelings, too. Any sadness you feel can soften your spirit.

THOUGHT FOR TODAY: I need not feel ashamed of any sadness I feel, and I trust it will yield to even greater joy.

Day 2

> *When my body began to curve*
> *like a river*
> *I loosened my hair and*
> *floated, head first,*
> *the long hair diffusing around me,*
> *strange undulations,*
> *seagrass,*
> *nipples like pebbles.*
> —SIV CEDERING FOX

When I was a little girl, I remember thinking pregnant women looked uncomfortable. Now I know how easily our bodies can accommodate a guest, "curving like a river."

When you are well centered in yourself, you are better able to resist the cultural message that only skinny young women are attractive. When your pregnant body feels noble, you feel beautiful. You know that whatever else may be going on in your life, you are doing the most important work in the world.

Many women in early pregnancy still get terribly tired and find that fatigue makes them more vulnerable to feelings of ugliness or inadequacy. However you can manage it, try to change your schedule so you can rest when you're tired. Your spirit deserves rest. If there ever was a time in your life when you deserve to feel beautiful, this is it.

THOUGHT FOR TODAY: I will work toward the letting go of useless images, and try to learn to float with my changes.

Day 3

It is so simple, the tattooer said. Little scars that carry you along, that leave you beautiful. This, you will never lose.
—Andrea Cohen

Some of your sadness may be a kind of mourning for your youthful body. It's natural in a culture where youth is so overvalued, to feel that this pregnancy will age you, mark you, render you less attractive. Yet what could be more beautiful than a healthy woman's body in bloom?

Some women have a horror of fat. When they become pregnant they dread the distortion of their bodies, the abdominal swelling, because it resembles fat. They are afraid of looking grotesque. Many of us allow our perception of beauty to be severely restricted, squeezed into what advertising images define. Our culture doesn't emphasize or appreciate the beauties of pregnancy; if we did, we might lament how soon they pass.

Some women never manage to feel beautiful during pregnancy; their hair and skin changes affect them badly, and they feel puffy and dulled. If this is true for you, remember the condition is temporary. Keep yourself as healthy as possible; the little scars will carry you along, will make you beautiful.

THOUGHT FOR TODAY: I may not feel beautiful, but I know this pregnancy can endow me with power and grace.

Day 4

> *I had eight birds hatcht in one nest,*
> *Four cocks there were, and Hens the rest,*
> *I nurst them up with pain and care,*
> *Nor cost, nor labour did I spare,*
> *Till at the last they felt their wing,*
> *Mounted the Trees, and learn'd to sing.*
> —ANNE BRADSTREET

One spring when I lived in a second-floor apartment, a nestful of young robins hatched in a tree outside my kitchen window. In the first few weeks, whenever I happened to look their way their beaks were stretched wide with what looked like desperate hunger. Then, within a minute or two, some adult bird would fly toward them with food in its beak.

At first they made no sound. Gradually, over the time they were in the nest, their cries got louder and louder. I think there were four of them, and when they cried in hunger no one could miss it; their need was imperative. Soon after they reached this stage of loudness, they flew out of the nest. I missed the exact moments of their fledging, but I could tell they were gone.

Although your baby has taken over your life completely, it is only a temporary visitor in your nest. Its needs will be imperative, and you want to be able to meet its needs without being totally controlled by them. You will need to seek a delicate balance.

THOUGHT FOR TODAY: I will take care to meet my own needs, for if mine are unfulfilled I won't be able to meet my baby's.

> *A life I didn't choose*
> *chose me: even*
> *my tools are the wrong ones*
> *for what I have to do.*
> —ADRIENNE RICH

Some women feel nauseated throughout their entire pregnancies. One friend of mine not only felt sick to her stomach the whole time, she had to spend most of the nine months in bed. Almost every pregnant woman has some days when she feels burdened by the child's presence, and some of us struggle with it constantly.

These weeks are terribly important for your baby's growth and development; it is basically a formed, recognizable human being—just unfinished. You may be afraid that when you feel unwell, it means there's something wrong with your baby. As long as you are living a healthy life, rest assured that your feelings of nausea or fatigue reflect your body's adjustments to pregnancy. In mild cases, perhaps you can reinterpret your sensations and teach yourself to think of nausea as your child's claim, rather than as a signal that something is amiss.

Because all pregnancies—and all women—are different, no one can really know the details of anyone else's discomfort or the sacrifices pregnancy may entail. Nurturing this new life can mean choosing to feel ill; you deserve a great deal of appreciation and support for your courage.

THOUGHT FOR TODAY: I must remember that I have been given the right tools for what I have to do.

Day 6

. . . this presence in my body is insistent, pulling me down below surface into deep water, warm earth water. Aware of my body. This presence stays with me always, quietly. I move in a dream of the presence, the earth of my body. Pregnant a month, two months. A long time. So now I find out what time is. The day comes around me like a coat. The sun is time.

—MARILYN KRYSL

Your whole life can deepen with this pregnancy, as you discover capacities you never knew you had. "Discovery" might not be the right word, since we aren't always consciously aware of the processes in which we're involved. "Intuition" might be better: at the end of each day your fatigue gives you the sense that your energies have performed mysterious, difficult tasks.

Time now is doubled for you: there's your time and your baby's time. Yet what feels like two lives, the life outside and the life within, is really just one life, your life. You may be blossoming like a garden, but you are still the same thinking, feeling, doing woman you were three months ago.

Each day represents a very large proportion of your baby's life; when you pay close attention to its development, time slows down for you. Wear the sun each day like a coat; it is a gift.

THOUGHT FOR TODAY: I can feel my body rooting deeper, but my spirit soars as high as ever—maybe higher.

Day 7

> *Behold and see*
> *What a great heap of grief lay hid in me,*
> *And how the red wild sparkles dimly burn*
> *Through the ashen greyness.*
> —ELIZABETH BARRETT BROWNING

Along with great joy in your pregnancy and anxiety for the future, you may find a "great heap of grief" that you never suspected before. Even women who are happy-go-lucky, who seldom get depressed and try not to dwell on negative things, may find that opening their hearts to the spiritual richness of pregnancy and birth opens them also to feelings of sorrow.

If anything should go wrong for your baby, that great heap of grief would be appropriate. What you are feeling may be sorrow for all the losses in life, all the broken connections, deaths, and sadnesses that even the happiest, healthiest person is acquainted with. And if nothing goes wrong—and it probably won't; the overwhelming majority of "missed" pregnancies don't make it this far—your newfound knowledge of grief can soften you toward others, toward your baby. Along with the ecstasy of creation you will gain a new understanding of pity and tenderness.

THOUGHT FOR TODAY: I will try to let grief flow through me. It is a feeling as natural and healthy as love.

Day 8

The human frame being what it is, heart, body and brain all mixed together, and not contained in separate compartments as they will be no doubt in another million years, a good dinner is of great importance. . . .

—VIRGINIA WOOLF

As important as what you eat is how you eat it. The most wonderful vitamins and fiber and polyunsaturated lipids won't truly nourish you if you don't enjoy them. Breakfast shouldn't be swallowed standing up in the kitchen; even if it's just fruit and a protein drink or a whole-grain muffin, you can respect yourself enough to give the meal some time and pleasure, with music, a pretty place mat, a favorite pottery mug.

Similarly, you can't just eat a carton of yogurt at your desk, in the car, or standing up at the counter and call it lunch. Maybe that's all you'll eat, but you owe yourself a break to enjoy it. A protein drink or a carton of yogurt can taste really good, if you let yourself enjoy their flavor and texture.

It may be hard for you to work up any enthusiasm at all for eating. Yet not only are you eating for two now, you're eating as your baby's mother. You may have stinted yourself for years, eating at your desk or on the run, but you can unlearn these disrespectful habits. How are you ever going to teach your child to enjoy healthy nourishment if you neglect your own enjoyment?

THOUGHT FOR TODAY: I can nourish my spirit along with my body, with pleasure as well as with food.

Day 9

For this thing the body needs
let me sing
for the supper,
for the kissing,
for the correct
      yes.

          —ANNE SEXTON

Most of us, unless we have had medical conditions that forced our awareness, hardly ever think about our wombs— until we become pregnant. And only two or three times in most women's lives does the uterus become really important. We know it's there, because of our menstrual cycle, but we take it for granted.

It is really a miracle, when you stop to think of it, this safe place where your child can grow in peace, protected and nourished until its time comes to be born. Your body is skillfully engineered for birthing and bearing, with this nurturing secret inside, marvelous and matter-of-fact.

The more you learn about pregnancy, about the body's chemistry and how accurately we synthesize the chemicals we need to stimulate our responses, the more clearly you can see how we are folded into the great overall plan of the universe.

THOUGHT FOR TODAY: My love for my body is twinned with faith in a wisdom greater than my own. I'll learn not to take for granted those things I can't see or understand.

Day 10

> *Mucus is a protection, a kind of love.*
> —JOHN BERGER

Over your cervix is a plug of mucus that prevents anything from entering your uterus while your baby is inside. It's an automatic protection for you both, this slippery substance that defends without harming.

The complicated beauty of our bodies *is* love—strong, soft, yielding, enduring. Our experience before we are born is of total warmth and protection, where all our needs are met. Ever after, when we search for love this is what we will mean.

Because we are moral and ethical creatures as well as emotional ones, when we search for love we will seek not only our own total fulfillment but that of our loved ones as well. As we want safety for ourselves in the love of others, we also want it for those we love.

The most spiritual love starts with the earliest and most physical, with our own infantile needs and desires, and our knowledge of kinship with one another. The highest love leads to self-forgetfulness, but to achieve it we first must know ourselves thoroughly.

THOUGHT FOR TODAY: I gain greater understanding of myself through contemplating my baby's growth. Reflection brings me closer to serenity.

Day 11

The children of the present generation will grow up accustomed to women doctors, respecting and trusting them.
—ELIZABETH BLACKWELL

Work and women have changed pretty radically since Elizabeth Blackwell opened the medical profession to women in the late nineteenth century. Women's work is just about anything these days: government, civil engineering, and doctoring as well as canning tomatoes, making curtains, and birthing babies. If your baby is a daughter, she'll grow up knowing there's really nothing she can't do.

Set against this rapid, profound change is the ancient pattern of pregnancy and birth. For years, science fiction has featured fantasies about how human reproduction will take place entirely in laboratories: Children will be conceived in test tubes, gestated in lab jars, and reared in state-run nurseries. Despite a handful of test-tube conceptions, however, produced by great advances in our scientific understanding of fertility, pregnancy as we've always known it seems to be as popular as ever.

Why not? It's safe, healthy, and often a pleasure. This experience connects you with women of all kinds, from all ages and conditions. Widened opportunities for women include the safe choice of motherhood.

THOUGHT FOR TODAY: All human endeavors deserve respect, and any work we choose to do is work to be proud of.

Day 12

*One thing certain is that we do not pay enough attention
enough of the time.*

—NAN SHIN

In these coming months you can learn how to meditate or
pray more deeply than you've ever done before. It's through
meditation and prayer that we come to pay "enough attention"
to what's important in our lives.

So much of ordinary existence is consumed in trivial
details that we sometimes do forget to pay attention to great
things—to our ideals, our profoundest desires. Since pregnancy connects you directly to the elemental forces of the
universe, you will be able to turn your mind to those things
that deserve your attention. Not the bills or laundry or a
dinner menu, but our place in the cosmos, the love that
surrounds us, the great force of life itself that has brought a
new life to your body.

These are unknowable things, yet attention turned toward them is always well directed. They are mysteries, and
contemplation of them refreshes the spirit.

THOUGHT FOR TODAY: My growing discipline in meditation will help me pay enough attention to the most important
questions.

Day 13

When you have
once had
a great joy
it lasts always. . . .
—TOVE DITLEVSEN

Pregnancy can put you in touch with the full range of your feelings. Your awareness of anxiety is expanded, as well as joy; your fears are vivid, and so are your desires. The important thing is to keep a balance.

Great joy can be with you always, if you choose. You can evoke the same triumph and pleasure that you felt as a child when you won a race or a spelling bee. Joy can be your way of perceiving the world, even on ordinary days. Even when things go wrong, planes are grounded, people fall ill, or bottles slip from your hands and break, your existence can be joyful from moment to moment.

It's the small things—the very beat of your baby's heart with yours, its swimming movements against you, your walk that rocks it, the circling of your blood—all these faithful gestures can earn great joy for you. Joy can be found in the simple and complex: the joy of learning, the joy of loving, the joy of good health, the joy of finding wildflowers in spring, or slipping into cool water on a hot day.

THOUGHT FOR TODAY: My deepest prayer for my baby is that the joy it brings me can belong to it as well.

Day 14

It was life that would give [our daughter] everything of consequence, life would shape her, not we. All we were good for was to make the introduction.

—HELEN HAYES

Your baby's introduction to life is going to continue over the next eighteen or twenty years, and you'll have plenty of practice. Even now, you can resolve never to hide things from your baby, and to do your best to call things by their right names. If we are introduced to life gently and straightforwardly, it's more likely to deal fairly with us.

After the early years, you and your partner have only a limited influence on how life shapes your child. But you can certainly give it a good start, well nourished and comfortably provided. Beyond this, you must surrender your own concerns and simply have faith that life's consequential gifts will be kindly given.

Life has already shaped your child; an unknowable combination of genetic and environmental influences has determined many patterns that will become part of its behavior. An unknown portion of its destiny has already been determined, and all you can do is make sure you don't stand in the way of its progress.

THOUGHT FOR TODAY: I will pray for the wisdom to help my child make good choices, and the detachment to let it grow in its own way.

Day 15

The moment of birth is a very important one for the child and for the mother; it is at this moment that the child acquires a power or an essence over which he has no control, although he can make use of it. . . . A supernatural essence that forever after connects the person born with certain forces in the world around him . . .

—Elizabeth Marshall Thomas

How do you want your child to be born? Most women say they want to be awake and aware. Many want the father to be present. They want a birth that is easy and natural, with as little interference as possible, and they want to be able to hold their babies as soon as they are born. At the same time, they want themselves and their babies to be safe and comfortable.

Some women seek out such birthing styles as giving birth in water, with soft music playing and people they love around them. But events move rapidly during birth, and in even the healthiest pregnancy unforeseen complications can arise. Cesarean section may turn out to be best for mother and baby, or intensive monitoring, either of which would involve hospital trappings, gowns, and anesthesia.

The moment of birth is important, but the decision is never entirely yours. Whatever happens will be for the best, in the large scheme of which each one of us sees only a small part.

THOUGHT FOR TODAY: I will work to achieve the serenity that lets me accept whatever happens.

Day 16

Sometimes, suddenly the old story overcomes us.
Time triumphs then
And lets down its hair—
Shadowy black,
Trailing like a willow.

—HSIUNG-HUNG

Pregnancy and birth are surrounded by many old stories in our culture, some of them sad and painful, some impossibly glorious, saccharine, or gruesome, some of them clearly absurd. One old story that doesn't often get told is how gracious this condition is.

It's a story very much about time. Time always triumphs; life is bound to time and change, growth and development. Yet with the serenity that comes from accepting the passage of time, grace can be yours through all the changes.

Even your baby, fresh and new as it will be at birth, will change in time and eventually grow old. All living things bud, bloom, and fade; what we call death is always a change into other kinds of being. Acceptance is the key to grace, and faith leads to serenity and acceptance.

THOUGHT FOR TODAY: I can squander my energy struggling with inevitable changes, or I can cooperate with them gracefully. Time is my ally, not my enemy.

Day 17

Each lighted boat had a dark sister ship that laid a net around it, enclosing the crowd of flickering fish that danced in the green water below the lighted prow. Gradually the two ships neared each other, the circular net drew in, and the catch was lifted up between them. I always thought of these two ships, the light and the dark, as life and death, working together.

—FREYA STARK

"The day my father died," a friend told me, "I found out I was pregnant. He'd been ill for a long time, and when my mother called with the sad news, I had some happiness to share with her. But our grieving for him colored it."

The good news tempered their sorrow, as well, I thought. That's life's complex texture: joy and grief come twisted together. What we call death is always a change into other forms; so is what we call birth. The life force drives male and female cells together, pushes ducklings and turtles out of their shells, and will pull your baby out of your body into the world. Life and death collaborate; these are the names we give to parts of the life process, its building-up and breaking-down.

So the emotions we associate with death, grief and sorrow, are the complements to joy, associated with it like the twin halves of our breath: in, out; darkness, brilliance; sorrow, joy. The pain of loss is balanced by joy in a new life.

THOUGHT FOR TODAY: If I can let go of old grief, I can begin to feel new happiness.

Day 18

[Cassandra] "sees" the future because she has the courage to see things as they really are in the present. She does not achieve this alone.

—CHRISTA WOLF

Many women feel that their pregnancy gifts them with a kind of prophecy. With the help of books and doctors, meditation and prayer, they are striving to see things as they really are in the present. You have an abstract knowledge of the future—of how your child will be born. You want to learn enough about the physiology of labor and birth so that you can enter this difficult task with the best preparation.

But to connect the present with the future requires a leap of faith. You may "know" that most of your baby's internal organs are developed, and that they are basically formed. But its emergence from your body as a live baby in the world may still seem like an impossible trick.

Perhaps the true prophets are always those among us who learn how to believe the impossible. Perhaps to see things as they really are always signals the ability to believe in other possibilities.

THOUGHT FOR TODAY: As far as my life is concerned, I will practice possibility-thinking; it's up to me to believe in my baby's future—and my own.

Day 19

O maybe it's bad to have a child now, I cried, feeling it leap inside me like a fish in clear water.

—MERIDEL LESUEUR

There is much frightening and depressing news: ozone depletion, overpopulation, AIDS, environmental poisons. To keep a healthy perspective on these horrors, think of the many centuries of war and famine the human race has survived, and the fact that our history has never been tranquil. Very few people have ever enjoyed anything like the health and comfort we take for granted today. Yes, there are terrible threats to our well-being, but this is probably the best time ever to have a child.

Any anxieties you feel for your baby can help you toward a deeper awareness of our human needs for peace and simplicity. The mistakes we make as a species can still be undone; lakes and rivers can be restored to relative purity; air can be made breathable once again. New life can leap in the womb, with reasonable certainty of living out a peaceful, fulfilled span of years.

THOUGHT FOR TODAY: An augmented consciousness is a gift I'll keep long after my baby's birth. Our family can work together on the tasks of greatest importance: the ongoing maintenance and repair of the world.

Day 20

Posterity has not been the country of women. What chance has the female storyteller had, making her way through closed gates to an alien city to an inhospitable audience in the town square of the patriarchy?

—LOUISE BERNIKOW

The great written stories of the past have been mostly men's stories of heroes, wars, and conquests. Most of the women in them have been tragic figures—abandoned queens, like Cleopatra and Dido; martyrs, like Joan of Arc and Mary, Queen of Scots; or villains, like Marie Antoinette and Mata Hari. But this is changing. Our history is beginning to be told through the mothers: Elizabeth Cady Stanton and Susan B. Anthony; Jane Addams of Hull House; Sojourner Truth, Ida B. Wells, Mary "Mother" Jones, and Mary McLeod Bethune.

Our culture is learning to value parenting, not just the birthing of children but also the nurturing of life that both women and men can provide. Your experience of pregnancy and mothering can teach you its value—perhaps you already know it. Caring for one another, for our children, our own parents, and the world, is heroism of a different sort from conquering enemies and winning battles. It takes a day-to-day courage and persistence, rather than terrific bursts of achievement.

Nurture is quiet; it doesn't call attention to itself. But nurture keeps the world in running order.

THOUGHT FOR TODAY: I can teach my child a new, more positive ideal of heroism.

> *The lion prowls the sky*
> *and shakes his tail for you.*
> *Pieces of moon*
> > *fly by my kitchen window.*
> > —KATHLEEN FRASER

Do you find that you take the world quite personally these days, like Dylan Thomas's Mrs. Organ Morgan in *Under Milk Wood*, who says, "And mind the sun wipes its feet before it comes in"? Every news story you read or broadcast you hear affects you personally. Perhaps you're eager for the world to be as good a place as your baby deserves. We want the world to be an appropriate place for our children, and we'll go to considerable lengths to make it so.

The world isn't separate from ourselves, or from our children. We're part of one another, and our best way of securing welcome is to be welcoming. If we deplore the amount of wealth our society devotes to weapons, or the number of homeless people, let us address this directly, in our own lives. Politics is personal, and the personal is political; everything we like or dislike about the way we live today bears some relation to the choices we make.

THOUGHT FOR TODAY: My wishes for my baby have awakened me from a narrow concern with my own life. Among other gifts, this pregnancy has given me the power to make choices for a better world.

Day 22

When you've achieved an intense, almost total communion with someone—which is rare, ultra-rare—when you've lived a real-life love story, in a word, you never really leave each other altogether: there's a neatly laid out compartment in your heart that no one else can fill.

—MONIQUE PROULX

"I've never been so in love with anyone as I am with this baby," a friend of mine said, when her firstborn was about three months old. I was a little shocked; I hadn't even thought about having children myself, yet, and I didn't know what she meant. The kid was cute, but how could she be *in love* with him?

Now that I know how children grow inside us, how intimately they are part of us, body, heart, mind, and spirit, I understand better how my friend felt—how a mother-child bond might be the kind of "real-life love story" that never ends. Your connection with your baby is surely going to be a powerful one. It's through your baby's early experience of intimacy with you and your partner that it will develop its own capacity for love—for love of itself, first, and then for love of others.

As your child grows up, you'll be less and less intimate partners. But you both will have had the experience of total communion, and its lessons can be yours forever.

THOUGHT FOR TODAY: This intimate, silent bond contains everything we will ever need to know about love. Through it I can discover selflessness as well as the profoundest self-love.

> *Who knows better than we,*
> *With the dark, dark bodies,*
> *What it means*
> *When April comes a-laughing and a-weeping*
> *Once again*
> *At our hearts?*
>
> —ANGELINA WELD GRIMKÉ

April is a metaphor for tender pain in many poems, often—as in this one—having to do with birth, with the coming-into-being of new creatures of all kinds. Whatever time of year your child is born, it can bring April into your heart.

We spend much of our lives avoiding pain, avoiding extremes of emotion, seeking tranquillity. Yet we know that for the sake of birth, we must surrender calm. You must allow yourself to be swept and buffeted by strong physical and emotional currents that may test the limits of your endurance.

Pregnancy makes different demands on women, but somehow we all rise to the occasion. We're never called to give more than we have; you may be surprised at your own strength and resiliency. The discomforts of pregnancy may torment you, but you can bear them one moment at a time. Few other occasions in our lives bring us such opportunities for self-discovery.

THOUGHT FOR TODAY: Just as the torrents of spring are followed by summer's bloom and autumn's harvest, my pregnancy and labor will be fruitful.

Day 24

> *You can make*
> *people, or you*
> *can unmake. You*
>
> *can do or you*
> *can undo.*
> —MAY SWENSON

The choice of when and whether to bear children is a basic freedom in our society, and you have made your choice—you're now in the business of making and doing. Worries or negative thoughts may occasionally chase each other through your mind, but you have voted for the continuation of the human race, with your whole self. The creation of a new life says that you believe in our human ability to live in peace and share our plenty.

Fertility can be slightly embarrassing to a sophisticated woman—it's so unsubtle, like an on-off switch. There is no way you can avoid announcing what used to be called an "interesting condition," though pregnancy is much happier and healthier than in the days when it was spoken of in whispered euphemisms. Since you've got it, you might as well flaunt it.

THOUGHT FOR TODAY: I can turn embarrassment into pride when I focus on the larger meaning of my pregnancy. My partner and I are demonstrating our faith in the human species.

Day 25

Oh little island,
How can you be so secure,
When countless great mountains
Have sunk in the sea?
—PING-HSIN

Your baby is as well protected as it's possible to be, given human anatomy. Your pelvic girdle of strong bone cradles it. It lives in a sac of fluid that absorbs normal impacts. Your blood and your immune system protect your child from infection. Most accidental shocks or falls can hardly affect it at all.

So your normal activities are safe to enjoy, although you should probably consult your doctor about such strenuous recreation as horseback riding, snorkeling, or skiing. Most likely you'll be told that until your center of gravity shifts noticeably, you can do anything you did before—assuming you didn't do anything foolhardy.

If you led an active life before you got pregnant, you're probably in such good shape that you can work and play normally. But sometimes pregnancy is fragile, and you may have to take it very easy for the next six months. Even if you have to go to bed for the duration, there are ways to exercise and keep reasonably fit. Life can be dangerous, but your child is a well-protected little island.

THOUGHT FOR TODAY: The same power that keeps birds in the air and flowers in the field is on our side. I'll pray for my child's safety and my strength.

Day 26

Children are an expensive luxury. They cost a lot to raise; they are late in getting to work, because of the long training they must have; and few parents get anything back from them.
—LYDIA KINGSMILL COMMANDER

If you expect your child to show up in the assets column on your profit-and-loss statement, you're setting yourself up for disappointment. Your child's value can't be computed in ordinary accounting terms; children can't be presented with a due bill at birth, and parents can't keep a running tab on their expenditures, because we all know this bond isn't a fiduciary one.

Yet parents often feel tempted to debit their children emotionally, to keep some private accounting of what they cost in care, in worry, in domestic disquiet. This temptation reflects our own need for emotional nurture. Some of us may feel stinted emotionally by our own parents, and we look to our children for recompense. As long as parents understand that they may feel these impossible desires, they can greet their children with the love and unconditional welcome they deserve.

You and your partner owe your child life and a responsible upbringing, and your child owes you nothing—nothing but its healthy development.

THOUGHT FOR TODAY: I will do my best to zero out our accounts continuously, so no expectations are laid on us, no setups for failure, shame, or guilt, and no resentments—only hope and love.

Day 27

*Little cat, are you as glad to have me to lie
upon
As I am to feel your fur under my hand?*
—AMY LOWELL

Rather than dwelling on all the things you are giving your baby, this is a good time to stop and reflect upon what you're getting—the reciprocity of this project. You'll be getting a new name: Mama or Mother or Mom. You'll be getting a completely new wardrobe, even though some of it may be borrowed from recently pregnant friends and relatives, and you will get a completely new sense of your body. You'll have a new public identity; total strangers will know an intimate fact about you, and you'll be proud and pleased.

You'll be getting to know your doctor or birth advisor; you'll be getting vitamin supplements and iron pills; later on, you'll probably be getting seats on buses and having doors opened for you. You're also gaining a new spiritual awareness, because this pregnancy is changing and augmenting your spirit. Not only is there a new life within your body, but the life you're leading is renewed.

THOUGHT FOR TODAY: I resolve to approach my new life with a grateful attitude.

Day 28

*Can I regard my pregnancy as anything but one long
festival? . . . I especially remember how at odd hours sleep
overwhelmed me and how I was seized again, as in my
infancy, by the need to sleep on the ground, on the grass, on
the sun-warmed hay. A unique and healthy craving.*

—COLETTE

You may not think of this as a long festival, and there may
not be much sun-warmed hay in your life, but many pregnant
women say they have never felt this kind of fatigue, this
urgent sleepiness. One woman expressed it as "getting several
messages daily to stop and rest because important work is
going on inside."

Your baby is growing fingers and toes. Soon it will have
eyelids. These little physical details must be difficult to make.
Remember, you are a partner in your baby's growth. Making
its body and spirit is your work, too.

Your baby is changing so rapidly, no wonder you're tired.
The hollow ball of cells that attached itself to your uterus
several weeks ago is now a sac filled with fluid. Your child's
tiny body has grown out from the place of attachment; there's
a placenta, now, that nourishes it.

Of course you'll take pride in your child's development;
but you're not alone in helping it grow. You may feel the
fatigue of the effort, but a higher power is also with you, every
step of the way.

THOUGHT FOR TODAY: My deepest resources of energy
and love are being called upon. I'll pray for the power to give
my all.

> *The birth-cry summoning*
> *out of the male, the father*
> *from the warm woman*
> *a mother in response.*
> —MURIEL RUKEYSER

We have no choice, in most cases, to be female or male; yet the roles of "woman" and "mother," "man" and "father," are constructed on the ground of our biological genders. They are social roles, yet they firmly print our sexual identities.

Your child deserves parents who understand their roles broadly. You may have grown up in a family where father was away all day, making a living, and the house belonged to mother. Or perhaps your mother worked outside the home as well as in it, and your father cooked and cleaned along with her. Perhaps your mother went out to work and your father stayed home.

You and your partner will work out your own individual adjustments to your jobs, your gender, and your parenting roles. Your child will learn that both of you work, and either of you might stay home. It will be cared for by two adult humans who share many qualities, none of them necessarily male or female but all of them nurturing.

THOUGHT FOR TODAY: My gender will enhance my life, not limit it, and my child will learn this liberation from me.

Day 30

There is nothing inevitable. The actions of the past operate at every instant and so, at every instant, does freedom.

—NAN SHIN

Your baby is like a mysterious package, mailed to you from an unknown address, inevitably on its way, due to arrive around a certain day. Its safe arrival is based on thousands of possibilities, open choices, some of them made in the past by your ancestors and some made freshly by you every day.

Basic choices were made long ago: your choice of work, for instance, or partner. You don't have to select most of your daily actions, yet if you don't reaffirm your choices, they become automatic. Your life becomes a sleepwalker's.

Try to become fully aware today of how you choose to carry your baby. These choices rest on prior choices made by you and others, many of them connected to your social class. Thanks to these prior choices, you have good things to eat, adequate shelter, suitable clothes, fulfilling work, refreshing play. You have a life in which you can choose to create new life.

THOUGHT FOR TODAY: I hope I have chosen so wisely in my life that my baby and I can both achieve a full expression of our potential.

> *The call is for belief,*
> *As once for doubt.*
> *The old firm picture wavers*
> *As if in water*
> *Like a thing off-centered . . .*
> —ABBIE HUSTON EVANS

Women have been struggling to free ourselves from old stereotypes of femininity. We're more than our bodies, and we proudly cultivate our minds and spirits. In pregnancy, when we find ourselves wholly involved in our bodies and their changes, the transition can be a shock. Our most basic self-image "wavers/As if in water"; the familiar attributes that give us our solid physical identity are changing, sometimes from one day to the next.

Faith in the rightness of our lives can ease us. If you find yourself resenting the prospect of gaining weight and changing shape, surrender your negative feelings. You may not be able to let them go once and for all; our resentments are tenacious. You may have to perform this act of surrender every day for a while, or even several times a day. Pregnancy and motherhood will change everything about you, and you're preparing to welcome these changes gladly.

Be gentle with yourself. Your feelings are strong, and you have a right to them. Surrender and acceptance are difficult achievements, and you'll get better at them with practice.

THOUGHT FOR TODAY: I believe in the rightness of my pregnancy, and I'll seek a strong belief among the changes and doubts that lie ahead.

THIS MONTH'S VISIT TO THE DOCTOR

Date:

Weight: Blood Pressure:

Weight Gain:

This Month's Signs of Pregnancy:

Changes in Eating:

Changes in Sleeping:

Changes in Activities/Energy Level:

Reflections:

Questions for Next Month's Visit:

Day 1

And Something's odd—within—
That person that I was—
And this One—do not feel the same—
Could it be Madness—this?
                    —EMILY DICKINSON

Your body has been sending out pregnancy hormones since the first month, keeping your baby safe, making sure it gets enough nourishment, and preparing it for birth. These powerful substances can make you feel wonderful, once the fatigue of early pregnancy has mostly gone, but they can also make you feel crazy. Some women say that you feel as though another person has invaded your body, speaking with your voice, gesturing with your hands.

Your dreams may be odd and disturbing, out of control. Another person is growing inside you, and you may not always enjoy that idea. It's common for pregnant women to fantasize that the baby they are carrying is a weird space alien, a parasite, a foreign growth. Even women who have longed for pregnancy can feel this strangeness. If you feel that "Something's odd—within—" be assured that this ambivalence is normal.

THOUGHT FOR TODAY: This is a powerful new experience, and of course I'm frightened at times. But whatever happens, my source of spiritual strength is available to me. I have an open line to help.

Day 2

Regret is an appalling waste of energy; you can't build on it; it's only good for wallowing in.

—KATHERINE MANSFIELD

In the very early days of pregnancy, you didn't know you were carrying a baby. You may have drunk wine and coffee; you may have taken some prescription pills, all at a time when your baby was most vulnerable. You probably stopped using potentially harmful substances as soon as you had even an inkling that you were pregnant, but some part of you may be telling yourself you should have given them up earlier. "I should have been more careful." Should, should, should.

Regret is useless for building anything. But how does one stop? First, forgive yourself; calm yourself, remind yourself that you're doing the best you can. Generations of women bore healthy children before scientists proved that alcohol and coffee could harm them. Your mother didn't know that coffee and tea were harmful; she might even have smoked cigarettes while she was pregnant, and you turned out all right. The only thing regret accomplishes is to make you feel bad, and why should you want that at this happy time?

THOUGHT FOR TODAY: I need all my energy for creative uses, so I'll choose not to consume it unproductively.

Day 3

In the pursuit of learning, every day something is
    acquired.
In the pursuit of Tao, every day something is dropped.

Less and less is done
Until nonaction is achieved.
When nothing is done, nothing is left undone.

The world is ruled by letting things take their course.
It cannot be ruled by interfering.

—TAO TE CHING

Tao means "the way." On the way to spiritual serenity, most of our assumptions and expectations should be dropped. This pregnancy will give you a good chance to let things take their course.

This drama is not under your direction. The less you do, the less you'll need to undo. Seeking to simplify your life will put you in tune with the natural course of things—"the way." In our technologically progressive lives, we are always in danger of forgetting simplicity.

A telephone-answering machine may seem to ease my life, but it really makes it more complex; if messages are recorded, I must keep track of them. Acquiring things is almost never the answer to a problem, any more than hair dye is the answer to gray hair. Acceptance is the answer; letting go is the answer.

THOUGHT FOR TODAY: Questions only need answers. I can simplify my life by accepting rather than questioning the changes I'm living through.

Day 4

I sit in a chariot
but I do not drive.
It is the horses
that hold the reins.
—AESCHYLUS

A hypnotist once came to an assembly at my high school. He asked for volunteers from the audience. I didn't think he could hypnotize me, and I was right (I later learned that *willingness* is almost always necessary for someone to enter a hypnotic state). I felt proud of my power, but also a little sad to think I might never succeed in relinquishing my strong will.

For this part of your life's journey, you definitely do not hold the reins. You have surrendered to the process of pregnancy, perhaps more completely than you have ever surrendered to anything. Your doctor or midwife isn't really in control; she may congratulate you on how well the process is going, but neither of you is in the driver's seat. You do your best to collaborate with pregnancy, nourishing and caring for it, glad to join forces with the creative energy of the universe.

THOUGHT FOR TODAY: My pregnancy belongs to a power much greater than myself. Gladly I surrender, traveling with my baby toward our destination.

Day 5

One window is all I need
one window onto a moment of consciousness, seeing, and
    silence.

—FORUGH FARROKHZAD

Sometime this month you will probably feel your baby move. You will feel a gentle elbow or knee bumping into you—from the inside. It is a strange feeling, yet somehow familiar. Not like being jostled by a stranger in a crowd; more intimate, more ordinary. Not at all an insult; almost a caress.

When this quickening happens, some women say their baby becomes real in a way it hadn't been before. You know many things about your baby because you've read them in books, or been told by your doctor or birth advisors; you know it's beginning to grow downy hair called lanugo all over its body, and that most of this will disappear before you ever see it. Feeling your baby quicken gives you a different kind of knowledge of its bones, its strength. It may only be six or seven inches long, but its muscles are active.

Quickening opens a window onto a new kind of consciousness. In silence you feel the ripples of your baby stretching to discover the limits of its world.

THOUGHT FOR TODAY: At these moments I realize that I am my baby's world; its limits are totally contained within me, and I am humbled.

Day 6

For me, conception, pregnancy, and birth are a conscious choice. I wouldn't want it any other way.

—GINGER EHRMAN

Being able to choose this pregnancy is a gift. Thanks to improved methods of contraception, women now have this choice with a considerable degree of certainty.

Many women have always had to juggle children and work, but middle- and upper-class women, professionals, scientists, artists, and scholars, usually had to choose between them, unless they were rich, well organized, and had cooperative husbands so they could schedule child care into their productive lives. For many of our foremothers, children were the center of life, and more than that—their life's work. It's easy to understand that most women were happy to choose the career of raising children over the kind of paid work that was available to them.

You have the good fortune to be able to choose both work and children. Bearing a child is the most important work anyone can do, but this pregnancy is enhancing all your capacities. Whatever you do in the future, you will be better at it because you have chosen to be a mother.

THOUGHT FOR TODAY: I'll be able to choose my own style of motherhood, and I trust myself to make the right choices.

Day 7

There has never been a period when education has trained women for the possibility of motherhood, and it is time that such training was begun.

—DORA RUSSELL

Did you receive any training for "the possibility of motherhood"? In one sense, your whole life has been preparation; you are certainly bringing to this experience all the richness you have accumulated in your life to date. But strictly speaking, few women have any training at all.

In grade school, sex education often amounts to no more than an incubator tray of chickens—fascinating, but not much practical use. In high school there are hygiene classes, which most of us giggled our way through. Maybe the boys learn something about menstruation; most girls don't hear anything they don't already know.

Nowadays, some high-school students are already parents, and they can bring their babies to day-care centers at their schools. These teenage mothers and fathers can take classes in child care and nutrition, and they are much better prepared than many. Of course, in some cases help given earlier would have enabled them to time parenthood more advantageously.

THOUGHT FOR TODAY: My baby's generation deserves more thoughtful preparation for parenting, and I'll do my best to see that they get it.

Day 8

I am that serpent-haunted cave
Whose navel breeds the fates of men.
All wisdom issues from a hole in the earth:
The gods form in my darkness, and dissolve again.
—KATHLEEN RAINE

The earliest people worshipped goddesses of fertility. Some of the oldest religious artifacts that have been found are little figures of pregnant women, with huge bellies, like the Venus of Willendorf. They're somewhat grotesque to our eyes, but we can understand the power of the images. Fertility is still a great mystery.

Scientists have a picture, now, of the hormonal cycles in which our bodies release the ova that meet the sperm to begin embryonic life, and successful research has made it possible for couples with reproductive difficulties to conceive and bear babies. Yet the flowering of a new body and spirit from the mating of two cells is still as wonderful and mysterious as it ever was.

In your own body, you can feel the power of the ancient knowledge that was attributed to serpents and to oracles. Superstition and belief, pagan awe and modern religious faith all celebrate the same mystery, the new life within.

THOUGHT FOR TODAY: The burgeoning of my body brings me close to the religious mysteries of all time. I am an incarnation of the ancient goddess.

Day 9

After all the work I'd done during my first trimester to stake out my own emotional territory, to define the experience of pregnancy in a personal way, the last words I expected to find myself writing in my journal were: "These days I feel so fulfilled, so contented."

—ROBERTA ISRAELOFF

Many women say that nothing in their lives makes them feel so utterly right as being pregnant—so *good*—not just well, but morally good, creative, productive, above reproach. After the fatigues and mild nauseas of the first trimester are behind them, many women also feel strong, energetic, and in tune with themselves.

Your baby has officially graduated from an embryo to a fetus. Its external reproductive organs have formed—although its sex was decided about eight weeks ago—and its fingernails are developing. Your breasts are growing bigger and so is your belly; many women find this makes them feel ripe and womanly. Your feeling of rightness matches your place in the grand design of life on the planet. It can be bliss to feel fully in tune with oneself, so content.

THOUGHT FOR TODAY: I am both proud and humble; meditation soothes the soul and keeps me connected to my source of spiritual strength.

> *It is the best thing.*
> *I should always like to be pregnant,*
>
> *Tummy thickening like a yogurt,*
> *Unbelievable flower.*
> —SANDRA MCPHERSON

Flowers are the reproductive organs of plants, showy and perfumed to attract the notice of the birds and insects that help them reproduce. Our culture downplays the connection between sexuality and birth, but many pregnant women feel it very strongly. Pregnancy is sexy; many pregnant women feel beautiful, like orchids; why don't we have extravagant maternity clothes that flaunt the swelling abdomen?

If you are feeling sexually powerful, it's a gift to be savored. Some women don't; pregnancy turns them off. Whether or not you feel your sexuality enhanced, your health and strength praise the source of life, and the child within you is a living prayer.

THOUGHT FOR TODAY: All the pleasures of my body are aspects of blessedness. I will be grateful for the strength and beauty I possess.

Day 11

Are there languages without words? Of course. We know there are, only our vanity keeps us from acknowledging them.
—FREDERICK LEBOYER

What LeBoyer calls our vanity might also be called our need for control. The wordless languages aren't always obedient to our will. The things we "say" with our bodies have to do with our most powerful, intimate states of feeling and of being. Babies' crying is one form of this wordless communication, like murmurs of love, or dancing, or the body language of fear and anxiety.

Sometimes adults are afraid that we won't understand our babies. A college professor told his pregnant wife, "I really don't understand children until they can talk to me."

But his wife thinks he'll do just fine. "He's anxious," she told me, "like all expectant fathers. This is the way he chooses to experience his anxiety."

With new babies, we must surrender to wordlessness. Sometimes adults use words to hide their feelings; we put up barriers of language between ourselves and others, we talk so as not to deal with our feelings. With a new baby, one doesn't have that option.

THOUGHT FOR TODAY: Love and faith will help me understand my child's wordless communication.

Day 12

When she was very small, my mother once settled herself in a basket of clean wash in imitation of a nesting robin, and was scolded by her mother for it. An only child like me, she made her paradise, her escape hatch, out of the nature around her.
—JOHN UPDIKE

Will your child be an only child? This charming picture of a little girl nestled in a basket of clean laundry gives a vivid sense of an only child's imagination. Only children are sometimes lonely, but having to make up much of their own play stimulates them to develop inner resources that often bear fruit in later life.

Whether or not your child ever has sisters or brothers, it will call on you for an understanding of its world at least equal to this son's understanding of his mother's. Would you scold your child for dirtying a pile of clean wash? (Of course, doing the laundry is easier now than it was for John Updike's grandmother.) Or would you be able to enter into the spirit of the robin's nest?

Staying in close touch with the child you were, who survives in your spirit, will help you to understand the child you carry in your body. And the spiritual sustenance you draw from your faith will protect you from loneliness.

THOUGHT FOR TODAY: I hope I can communicate my faith and spirit to my child so it will never be lonely, whatever solitude its life may hold.

> *It happens*
> *only when you give it*
> *room. That milky beast.*
> *Fed on the chance that it might be,*
> *it is.*
> —SHIRLEY KAUFMAN

Your circulatory system is adding inches, feet, yards of blood vessels to nourish the new spaces in your body. Your breasts are growing larger, richer, and more complex. Perhaps you can feel the coordination of belly and breasts; the nerves in your nipples, when stimulated by your baby's sucking, will cause your uterus to contract and help it to return to its prepregnant state. Many women thrill to the knowledge that their body creates food that will nourish the baby growing inside them, but some have difficulty reconciling their erotic feelings about their breasts with the nurture of breast-feeding.

Because in our culture breasts are so fetishized, glorified, and depersonalized, it may come as a shock to realize that they're a superbly efficient means of nourishing human offspring; they will give pleasure to your baby, too, along with nourishment.

THOUGHT FOR TODAY: I don't have to separate my sexual feelings from my nurturing feelings. I'll take pleasure in sharing my body's richness.

Day 14

It has never yet been a world right for love, for those we love, for ourselves, for flowered human life.

—TILLIE OLSEN

Sometimes I imagine a better world, one where wealth is shared more equally so that no one must live in want. Where science and technology work together with the environment, not trying to exploit it for quick profits but cooperating so that plants, animals, and people are all respected, all deemed worthy of survival.

In this dream world, drug dependency and other diseases are rare misfortunes, and crime is almost unknown. Peace is studied in all the schools, and those who are elected to govern are the women and men who are the most skilled at resolving conflicts peacefully. In this world, every bud can flower.

Your baby is coming into a different world, yet it contains the seeds of that dream. You can teach your baby what you have learned in your life about bringing into being a world where human possibilities are valued. Perhaps your child's generation will succeed in the struggle to bring about our world's rebirth.

THOUGHT FOR TODAY: I want so much for my child. The most precious gift I can bestow is my sense of possibility.

I am a woman giving birth to myself.
—ANONYMOUS

People toss around the terms "born again" or "rebirth" as though once didn't quite do it. All of us can give birth to ourselves many times over in our lives. Every stage in a person's growth has something of rebirth about it, including some pain at giving up an earlier stage. At every stage there's also the joy of arriving and bewilderment about how one got there.

When we encounter people who seem frozen, or stuck, we may sense that they fear the pain of a rebirth more than they long for the enlightenment. Something in their lives prevents them from growing into a new consciousness or understanding.

Nowadays, when birth occupies a certain proportion of your waking thoughts, your own inner growth may seem less important than your child's physical growth. Nonetheless, your share of this partnership is to continue giving birth to yourself. We keep on growing our whole lives; your growth into motherhood will coincide with your child's first birth.

THOUGHT FOR TODAY: I pray for courage to overcome fear of rebirth, and to be strengthened in all that I do.

Day 16

There is a point with me in matters of any size, when I must absolutely have encouragement as much as crops rain; afterwards I am independent.

—GERARD MANLEY HOPKINS

You are well into your second trimester, embarked on a matter of considerable size and importance, yet you probably aren't visibly pregnant. There isn't much cultural support for your current stage of life. Some women respond to this sense of being marginal by telling everyone they know—sometimes even strangers—about their pregnancy. This need to tell people may be a signal that you're at a point where you need encouragement.

Other women respond by not telling anyone, almost seeming to forget that they are pregnant at all. In a month or two, they tell themselves, I'll wear maternity clothes, and everyone will know. But this can be a lonely adjustment.

Since, in our culture, a little thing like early pregnancy goes unnoticed, you have to valorize your condition all by yourself. Never forget that your support is always available. Your spirit deserves refreshment and reaffirmation, for you are on a path that leads to great achievement.

THOUGHT FOR TODAY: I deserve praise. Great work demands great effort, and great encouragement.

Day 17

It is precisely for feeling that one needs time, and not for thought. Thought is a flash of lightning, feeling is a ray from the most distant of stars.

—MARINA TSVETAEVA

In order to grow up, we had to learn to stifle our feelings. Everyone does; your child will, too. It's just not possible to live in society with the naked feelings we're born with. We learn to transform, conceal, and dilute our feelings, just as we learn to eat with utensils and to wear clothes.

As adults, we can think rapidly but we may not always know how we feel. Sometimes we need to take time—time to meditate, to dive deep within ourselves and bring up crusted pearls of remembered feeling.

Your feeling self may be closer at hand, these days. Many women find that tenderness and anger, fear and desire, are very close to the surface during pregnancy, and the nearness of these emotions can be both delightful and alarming. You may feel out of control, especially if you customarily present a rather calm exterior.

There is no cause for alarm. Your feelings can't harm you, no matter how strong they are. You can let them flow through you, experience them, and let them go. Everything changes; the anguish in our lives has no more staying power than the bliss—unless we cling to it.

THOUGHT FOR TODAY: Wouldn't it be wonderful if I could always keep my feelings close at hand? Another gift of pregnancy.

Day 18

We were standing beneath a great cottonwood tree that leaned green over us like a mother. Yes, she said, putting her hands on my shoulders, a new heart is growing.

—MERIDEL LeSUEUR

Your baby's heartbeat can be heard about now. Such convincing evidence of life! Also in this month, your child's bones have hardened from cartilage into dense, hollow calcium structures. They have developed bone marrow, which has begun to make blood cells. Blood circulates through the fetal heart, which beats strongly and rapidly, almost twice as fast as yours.

A new heart: In our culture *heart* stands for so many things: courage, sincerity, loyalty, pity, and love. We use it to mean deep feeling, the feeling core of a person. Someone cold and unsympathetic we call *heartless*. So your child's growing heart means more than just a pump for its fresh blood; it signifies that the new life belongs to an ally, someone who will be on your side. Whatever feelings are in your heart, you can share them with your baby, and miraculously they'll be increased.

THOUGHT FOR TODAY: New heart, I think of you as my friend. And I am yours.

Day 19

. . . music is able to simulate that state when the infant still feels itself to be coextensive with the mother's body, a state in which all sensation appears to be authentic—before the alienating social codes of language and culture intervene, before one is even aware of being an individual separate from the mother.

—SUSAN McCLARY

Our response to music is more immediate than to other kinds of expression, even if we ourselves are trained musicians. Certain strains of music can evoke certain feelings—sensuality, gaiety, gloom—as certain colors can, purely and simply.

A new father bathed his baby girl on the first day after her birth, and she lay relaxed in his arms, not fighting the strange experience. A nurse, observing them, said, "She recognizes your voice."

When you hear music, your baby hears music; when you and your partner talk, your baby will hear your voices, really hear them—learn to know them so well that it will recognize you anywhere, even in the birthing room.

Music takes us back to our own infancy. I used to think maybe I'd heard some Beethoven symphonies in utero, because I loved them even as a small child. Music is like fluid love; it will form a bond between you and your child, just as your birth fluids do.

THOUGHT FOR TODAY: To the rhythm of my heartbeat and the music of our voices, I'll add more music, to welcome my child into the world.

Day 20

> . . . *thou art Being and Breath*
> *And what thou art may never be destroyed.*
> —EMILY BRONTË

Pregnant women sometimes dream that their pregnancy itself is a dream. You may dream that you wake up to find you have your period. Then you wake up and find that the dream has been an anxious fantasy.

What are the ways in which your child is real to you? First was the evidence of the missed period; then the early physical feelings—perhaps nausea and fatigue, nipple tenderness, changes in appetite, distaste for certain smells. Then the first prenatal visit to your doctor or nurse who looked at your cervix, peered into your eyes, and took your blood. Then the test result: positive! Then the sonogram, seeing a funny outline of your baby, like a child's follow-the-dots picture. And now, of course, it has quickened.

But more than all these is the emotional connection you can feel with your baby—the idea of it, its spirit. This precious bond can't be measured physically. You will never hold an image of it in your hand. Yet it's there, as surely as your baby's heartbeat, and it will connect you forever, no matter what the future may hold.

THOUGHT FOR TODAY: Our bond may be intangible, but it is nonetheless real.

Day 21

She was like someone standing before a great show window full of beautiful and costly things, deciding which she will order. She understands that they will not all be delivered immediately, but one by one they will arrive at her door.

—WILLA CATHER

What a metaphor for life—a display window full of "beautiful and costly things"! When you feel especially chaotic, out of control, you need to remind yourself that the confusion is made of many pieces of good fortune: your health, your baby's health, your work, relationships, home. You have a profusion of beautiful things in your life, but they all have cost you something: time, effort, emotional energy. And your baby, however precious and wanted, is literally costing you flesh, blood, and breath.

The different acquisitions in your life may not all appear at once, but one by one they will arrive at your door, taking their place in the development of your family's story. For now and for the future, remember that in life, what you get is always worth the price you pay for it. Happily, your baby will be delivered to you before very long, and you'll have a lifetime to appreciate its beautiful and costly attributes.

THOUGHT FOR TODAY: My physical and emotional resources are more than equal to the demands placed on them. I can love my child unconditionally.

Day 22

In the kitchen, the old cat, stunned by
*   time,*
tightened into a ball. I sat, surrounded by all the
*   things*
I hadn't done, surprised by my life.
—CAROLYN MILLER

It's probably a good thing to be surprised by one's life from time to time. Many of us go from day to day almost automatically, without reflecting on or savoring the myriad qualities of our experience. Pregnancy for many women slows down the pace of life, allowing them time for surprise.

It may surprise you, for example, that you feel both proud and secretive about your pregnancy. If a stranger were to ask whether you are pregnant, you might feel a little insulted, in spite of your desire for recognition, or invaded, as though the question crossed some boundary of your privacy. It's your secret—although within a short time everyone who sees you will know it.

This little complication of feelings might surprise you. Of course you're proud; of course you want to tell the world. But you want to do the telling, you don't want to be public property. This is your achievement, and while you claim credit for it you'd probably also like a little delicacy, a little acknowledgment of your privacy.

THOUGHT FOR TODAY: I can be proud one day and reticent the next. I will accept and savor these small ways in which my life surprises me.

> *Every hour, every moment*
> *has its specific attendant Spirit . . .*
> —H. D.

In many religions there are schedules of devotions; orthodox Jews and Muslims say prayers before washing and before cooking. There are prayers for work, for rest, and for love. Nuns and monks have scheduled hours of prayer. Buddhist communities welcome each day with prayers for its holiness. Time, which sometimes seems to drag if we don't make ourselves conscious of it, is really made up of many small sacrednesses. Every moment has its spirit, and all are holy.

Your connection with your baby is of the most sacred kind. You are the mystery of life itself, the two of you together, sharing one body now and preparing to become two. Can you make yourself aware of each moment, as it blesses you?

Probably not, realistically speaking; most of us are too immersed in the swim of our ordinary days, working and playing, shopping and talking and caring for ourselves. But this adventure asks you to claim some space within your life for extra consciousness, extra awareness. To renew your sense of wonder and your knowledge that your process is a prayer in itself.

THOUGHT FOR TODAY: As pregnancy progresses, my connection to my baby grows and deepens, giving me rich material for reflection.

Day 24

"Oh! mothers aren't fair—I mean it's not fair of nature to weigh us down with them and yet expect us to be our own true selves. The handicap's too great. All those months, when the same blood's running through two sets of veins—there's no getting away from that, ever after."
—HENRY HANDEL RICHARDSON

Fairness is an idea we apply to relations between people. How funny to expect it of nature. It isn't *fair* for trout to eat mosquitoes, nor rivers to flood, nor cabbage worms to munch our garden plants; it just is.

Mother-child relations, at least in pregnancy, just are. Nothing fair about them; your baby lives comfortably inside you, nourished and maintained by your body. And what do you get in return? Discomforts, anxieties—and joy, serene, soaring joy, happiness of a kind you never imagined before.

Of course, the same blood doesn't flow between you. Your child has had its own blood from the start. You exchange nutrients and wastes through the delicate membrane barrier, first in the chorionic villi and then in the placenta, but your bloods stay separate. So do your hearts and your spirits, unless you deliberately enmesh them. The love between you will be enhanced when you can respect your separateness as well as your closeness.

THOUGHT FOR TODAY: I can dwell on the unfairness of life, or I can celebrate its variousness. It's something I can't control, so I will choose to honor the differences and find joy in them.

Day 25

There is one great thing, the only thing, to live to see the great day dawning.

—INUIT SONG

Children give us a kind of immortality. Part of you will live on in your child; and that part will be able to see the future. Of course the germs of you that your child will carry forward into generations yet to come won't include your eyes, ears, and consciousness; if that great day dawns, "you" probably won't be around to see it. But the wonderful toughness and persistence of this verse says, We're going to hang on until we make it.

This hopeful toughness is something you can pass on to your child. The courage to survive is noble, worth nurturing and celebrating. That spark is truly immortal; it passed to you from your ancestors, and your child can transmit it to all your descendants.

You can communicate it to others as well, whether or not they are in your family line. Hope is even more contagious than despair, because hope is coded into our bodies; life itself tells us to survive, to hang on, to live until the great day dawns, and others welcome our encouragement.

THOUGHT FOR TODAY: Each day is another step toward the great day. I will pledge myself to celebrate its coming.

> *I cannot sing the old songs now!*
> *It is not that I deem them low;*
> *'Tis that I can't remember how*
> *They go.*
> —C. S. CALVERLEY

Every once in a while, we come to a watershed in our lives: a place after which everything is different. Often pregnancy is such a place. You are the same person you were four months ago, but that person may seem quite remote— almost as distant as your earlier selves, the eager first grader or the adolescent anxiously waiting for her first menstrual period.

Different things seem important to you now; you may forget how the old tunes go. Thoughts of birth, babies, and children may occupy your consciousness. When you think about movies you saw last year, or books you've read more recently still, what you remember about them are the mother-child connections.

Pregnancy changes your outlook on the world. It is exciting to see how we are changed by life's profoundest experiences, but it's only human to miss, sometimes, our earlier selves—the woman who remembered the romantic scenes and not the maternal ones; whose thoughts were occupied by adults rather than babies. No doubt a time will come in your life when that's appropriate again, another watershed.

THOUGHT FOR TODAY: Everything in life has its season. I will flow with my changes, serene in the knowledge that this too will change.

". . . somehow it was like I had been born again. Maybe that's what gives a woman strength when she finds out she's pregnant. At least some part of her will go on."

—ANN CORNELISEN

Many students of social policy have written that poor women are not motivated to prevent pregnancies, even though having more children may make them even poorer, because they feel so well, so hopeful when they are pregnant. Pregnancy does make one feel strong and equal to life's challenges, as well as protected by a powerful hope. The southern Italian peasant women that Ann Cornelisen writes about live in desperate poverty, yet they cherish these feelings of strength and hope.

You and your child are fortunate in the relative comfort and security of your lives. You have enough, and more than enough; you live in a rich country and your families are secure and prosperous enough to afford you the advantages of good nutrition and shelter, education, medical care, healthy recreation.

It seems cruel that only in repeated pregnancies can some women find comfort to bear the misery of their lives; for those pregnancies will result in more mouths to feed, more bodies to clothe, ultimately more misery.

THOUGHT FOR TODAY: My best hope for my child is not just material comfort, but my spiritual gifts as well.

Day 28

Gather into yourself
like a bee
the hours that fall open
under the bright shaft of the sun
ripening in heat,
store them

and make of them
   honey days.
      —NUALA NI DHOMHNAILL

Can you keep the bright, sweet hours and use them for nourishment when life seems bleak or dull? Now would be a good time to develop that skill, if you can, so you can teach your baby. The good times, loving, open, and joyous, teach us to blossom. Perhaps if you can grasp this lesson well enough, you can become the sort of person who carries her own sunshine, lightens her own clouds.

All experiences are useful, not just the happy ones. Pain and sadness soften us and teach us humility. The best lesson is to distill all experience, letting go of what you cannot use and treasuring what you can; letting go of bitterness or resentment, of vanity and ego-tripping, and holding on to patience, wisdom, joy.

THOUGHT FOR TODAY: Honey is the distilled sweetness of a bee's lifetime of labor. I can dedicate myself to distilling sweetness from my life, to nourish my child.

Day 29

As the annual cycle of life unfolds through the sequence of seasons, the various directions, and their people and attributes, each in turn comes to play the central and dominant role. Each is meaningless except as it contributes to the whole.
—SAM D. GILL

The four directions, north, south, east, and west, are important in native American Indian religions; ceremonies begin with an invocation to the four directions, and all aspects of life are associated with them. In these integrated, relational systems of belief, spirits and attributes are not fixed but exist in relation to one another.

Your baby can help you think in more relational, holistic ways. When you read or hear of scientific discoveries or political events, you can relate them to the kind of world you want for your child. Nothing is entirely good or bad in itself; its worth depends on how it will affect people's lives.

The four directions blend into one another in a continuous harmony—their winds, their seasons, their plants and animals. Anything we invent or add to them becomes a part of many systems.

THOUGHT FOR TODAY: My baby's life will be a continuous web of relationships, and I can help foster this bonding process.

Day 30

For women to assert as equals their needs in the bedroom required a sense of equality that had to pervade the kitchen, nursery, and study as well. . . .

—LINDA GORDON

A grandmother came to visit her new great-grand-daughter in the hospital. Her grandson-in-law was changing the baby's diaper, and the old woman was shocked. "Don't!" she said. "You'll spoil her."

"Spoil her, Nana?" said her granddaughter.

"Not her! You!"

At first the new mother and her husband were ruffled by this assumption; then they laughed. Then they were able to talk about it with the grandmother, and by the end of the visit she acknowledged, "I think I was a little jealous. Your grandpa would never have done such a thing."

How lucky you are to be living at a time when fathers gladly share the tasks of caring for their children. You may choose to return to the labor market when your child is six months old, or a year, or you may want to work full time inside the home—"Every Mother Is a Working Mother!"—but wherever you work, you and your baby's father can share equally in its upbringing. Hopefully, by the time your child has children of its own, they won't even understand this story.

THOUGHT FOR TODAY: Liberation begins with freedom from stereotyped thinking. This freedom is another one of my gifts to my child.

Day 31

After spending a week reading creation myths, I began to study pictures of the reproductive system, looking for parallels in iconography. Needless to say, they were there— macrocosmic and microcosmic reflections of the creation and life processes, just as I had suspected. A nova looks just like an ovum, and the oceans on the earth's surface make patterns like nerve cells.

—JUDY CHICAGO

When the first satellite photos of the earth's surface were published, many people were moved by their beauty, and by the familiarity of the images. The entire planet looks like an egg yolk or a baby's head, soft, yielding, and rich with possibilities.

It should not surprise us to find the shapes and forms of life reflecting the same rhythms of integrity and interconnection, from scanning electron micrographs of single cells to survey maps and aerial scans. The long roots of our nerves branch like willow trees or the tributaries of a river basin. Crystal-like branchings appear in cervical mucus, in snowflakes, in diamonds. Our world is an organic world, and we're inscribed within it as it is formed within our minds and spirits. Our shapes are the shapes of life itself.

THOUGHT FOR TODAY: My baby and I are living beings that extend backward and forward in time and space, throughout the history of the universe.

THIS MONTH'S VISIT TO THE DOCTOR

Date:

Weight: Blood Pressure:

Weight Gain:

This Month's Signs of Pregnancy:

Changes in Eating:

Changes in Sleeping:

Changes in Activities/Energy Level:

Reflections:

Questions for Next Month's Visit:

Day 1

Some people think doctors and nurses can put scrambled eggs back in the shell.

—DOROTHY CANFIELD FISHER

My aunt took very literally the diet sheet that her doctor gave her to guide her nutrition during pregnancy. She consulted it every evening, and if she hadn't eaten everything on the sheet during the day, she ate it before she went to bed. If the instructions said a cup of cottage cheese and she'd only eaten half a cup that day, she'd eat the rest, although she hated cottage cheese; if it said two servings of a vegetable and she'd only eaten one, she conscientiously ate the other, standing up in her clean dark kitchen.

My aunt totally gave over her independence of judgment. To some extent that may be good; we all need to be able to follow "doctors' orders." But surely, she could have had the same nutritional value from foods she enjoyed!

We choose our doctors and advisors for their skill and wisdom, but as patients we don't need to give away our powers of choice or reasoning. If a nurse or doctor makes a suggestion you don't agree with, or don't understand, ask for clarification; don't just nod or let it go. You deserve respect, too.

THOUGHT FOR TODAY: Clear communication and understanding are an essential part of health care.

Day 2

I have just realized that the stakes are myself
I have no other
ransom money, nothing to break or barter but my life
my spirit measured out, in bits . . .
—DIANE DIPRIMA

Sometimes a pregnant woman feels very alone in this great venture, solely responsible for her baby. Not just its growth—for which she *must* take responsibility—but also its entire future, its being, its thoughts and actions, its soul. But you are not alone; just as you have your own source of spiritual nurture that gives you serenity and strength to lead your life creatively, with hope, so your baby has its own very special connection to a power greater than itself.

While you and your baby share one body, it is your spiritual companion as well as your constant guest. But the baby is and will be its own person. Your duty toward it is one of love, not domination; you will learn at least as much as you teach.

Your happiness is assured when you surrender control to that higher power that guides your destiny with a wisdom greater than any mortal's. You and your baby are loved, and the love you'll feel toward one another will nourish and not deplete you.

THOUGHT FOR TODAY: My baby and I are growing as we were meant to grow, with the best possible guidance.

Day 3

*. . . I had been caught short by how sexual I felt. . . . The
pleasure of no birth control was only part of the story. So
were hormones. I was in a nearly continual state of excitement, wanting to make love every day, several times a day,
and at odd hours, like a kid.*

—ROBERTA ISRAELOFF

Pregnant women usually aren't thought of as sexy in our
culture, yet they are—*you* are—undeniably attractive. You
may feel like a fertility goddess, and your partner may
welcome this new sensuality in your relationship.

But it may be that your glorious fecund shape does not
turn your partner on. There may be uncomfortable echoes of
your partner's own mother, or other powerful taboo feelings.
When you want to revel in your sexuality, you may be
awakening some very unerotic responses.

You can still love and honor your burgeoning body, with
creams and lotions, pillows, music, perfume. Everything
changes; any erotic relationship goes through times of ebb and
flow. Don't let negative feelings cloud your serenity.

THOUGHT FOR TODAY: Relationships may change temporarily, but your pleasure in yourself can be stronger than ever.

What matters it that all around
Danger and grief and darkness lie,
If but within our bosom's bound
We hold a bright unsullied sky?
　　　　　　　—EMILY BRONTË

It may be hard for you to take seriously any bleak news from outside, when all within seems to be blessedly secure. Yet your baby is going to be born into this world, and the problems that our society sloughs off right now are problems your child's generation will inherit.

Rather than spending your time and energy on anything else, you may want to hold on to your wonderful feeling of assured safety that comes from good health and a strong faith in the rightness of life. That buoyancy and confidence ought to be shared by everyone.

After your baby is born, you can teach it concern. Along with well-child health care you can foster well-world attitudes, the deep ecological concern that will help your baby's generation save its world. Together you can learn what to do to help make this a world where everyone feels as safe as a baby in the womb, and as peacefully, happily creative as its mother.

THOUGHT FOR TODAY: My baby inspires me to think globally. I must learn to act locally.

Day 5

Today, like every other day, we wake up empty and scared.
Don't open the door to the study and begin reading.
Take down the dulcimer.

Let the beauty we love be what we do.
There are a hundred ways to kneel and kiss the ground.
—RUMI

As you come near to the midpoint of your pregnancy, remember that it's possible to pray in many different ways. Sometimes one feels holy while doing utterly mundane things—watching for birds or making love or just walking down the street smelling the sweet odors of the season. Your healthy body, your healthy pregnancy, is like a prayer in itself, because it praises the source of life and love. When you practice deep breathing, you can feel the rich blood flowing through your body. Each tiny muscle rejoices in its well-being.

Many women are wearing maternity clothes by this point in their pregnancies, whether or not they need the extra fabric for comfort. It's exciting to wear this special wardrobe, even if most of it is borrowed from friends and relatives. Big clothes are a badge of your honorable condition, and you deserve to wear them with pride. Think of them as your robes of office.

THOUGHT FOR TODAY: Holiness is where you find it, and it can be found wherever you look.

Day 6

There is too much fathering going on just now and there is no doubt about it fathers are depressing.

—Gertrude Stein

Stein wrote these words on the eve of the Second World War, and the scorn she heaps on "fathers" needs to be understood as meaning the heads of state, whom she saw rushing headlong into war. Such militaristic "fathers," who risk the futures of their sons and daughters, are indeed depressing. In all the millennia of human history, they haven't figured out how to resolve disputes over territory, religion, or ideology without sacrificing the young. These patriarchs oppress both men and women. Such "fathers" are the opposite of nurturing parents, male or female.

Later generations are escaping from these old, violent meanings of fatherhood; we're discovering that peace is a far more glorious study than war, demanding greater skill and yielding richer rewards. Your baby's father will probably complement you in caring for it, and your child will learn that true parents are concerned with fostering life.

THOUGHT FOR TODAY: I will practice peace, in the hope that my child's generation learns to resolve conflict peaceably.

Day 7

> *The art of losing isn't hard to master;*
> *so many things seem filled with the intent*
> *to be lost that their loss is no disaster.*
> —ELIZABETH BISHOP

Near the halfway point, pregnancy seems wonderfully solid. Any worries you may have had about losing your baby are past; it's moving, you can hear its heartbeat, and most women feel strong and healthy. Some mothers can even feel their babies hiccuping.

Your baby still has freedom to move, to turn around. It moves to your rhythm. Your pregnant body now is like a close pair of dancers, both of you following the same beat. Hard to believe this closeness will end with two creatures following separate paths—but it will.

The loss of this intimacy is no "disaster"; it's normal and necessary. Feeling so close to another being, the privilege of sharing one body, is a unique experience that can't be extended into life after birth. That close relationship is filled with the intent to be lost; it's one stage in an ongoing process, that gives way to the next stage.

THOUGHT FOR TODAY: Rather than losing closeness, I'll concentrate on what I will be gaining after my baby is born.

Day 8

The time to start worrying is when neither words nor experiences are new any longer. How many times can you breathe this breath?

—NAN SHIN

Every breath is unique; each moment greets us with new possibilities. To bring worries from the past into the present is to deny the freshness of life.

Each breath can only be taken once into your lungs, but it nourishes mother and baby together. The infant receives oxygen diffused from the mother's blood across the placental membranes, into its delicate new circulation. Each breath comes only once.

Each kick or flutter or hiccup comes only once, though you may come to expect them. They grow familiar, but you can keep that first true response in the back of your mind; each is as wonderful as the first movement you ever felt. Perhaps you cannot recapture awe every day, but don't let any of these precious signs become ordinary. Though pregnancy seems long, it's really only a short interlude in your life, and everything about it can be savored for the miracle it is.

THOUGHT FOR TODAY: Every moment of life—even those that seem to be repeated experiences—can be treasured when I know how to greet each day with gratitude for its freshness.

Day 9

When the pale apples are ready   then we return
the core to earth   after frost the late apples
redden   grow tart with time and the cold
  nights   we look west
toward the valley villages   the small orchard   the
  fruit
early and late tumbled under light snow
sweet mulch of this sweet earth

—GRACE PALEY

In some societies, the birth membranes are buried, after a baby's birth, under the threshold of the family's house—a symbol of how all things return to the earth. The compost heap or mulch pile is a vivid image for this cycle of birth and return. In other societies, the mother eats the placenta, perhaps to signal her renewal after the loss of the birth, perhaps as a way of taking back some of the nutrients her body has poured into the pregnancy.

Spiritual cycles are more hidden than physical ones, yet many people believe new babies come into the world with old souls. In Hindu philosophy, the souls of people and animals obey similar laws and return after bodily death in new shapes according to the progress each has made in previous lives. Existence is seen as a great wheel of time, in which life constantly flourishes, perishes, and provides occasion for new life.

THOUGHT FOR TODAY: I will honor the spirit that nourishes my baby, brand-new or reborn.

Day 10

> *O my floating life*
>
> *Do not save love*
> *for things*
>
> > *Throw* things
> > *to the flood*
> > —LORINE NIEDECKER

Being pregnant is a gloriously fleshly condition. Many women find they have never enjoyed their bodies more, the sheer physical pleasure of living. This is true even when the swelling belly makes things a bit awkward. As you journey through the next few months, you may grow even more awkward, yet the more of you there is, the more there is to enjoy.

For some women, this abundance is never pleasurable. They feel drab and ungainly the whole time, even when family and friends tell them how well they're looking. Although they stay healthy, they never feel well; they experience pregnancy as others experience an allergy.

If you're feeling like this, your compensation will be your increased spiritual awareness. Nourish your sense of humor; your connection to the universal source of love is illuminated by the invisible cord that joins you to your baby and to all creative energy.

THOUGHT FOR TODAY: What is truly important is not the flesh alone, whether that be enjoyed or just tolerated, but the current of spiritual energy that blesses you.

Day 11

People welcome true ideas.
—ELIZABETH BLACKWELL

No word in our language looks so clear and turns out to be so complicated as that little word *truth*. Blood has been spilled over it. To Elizabeth Blackwell, the first woman to graduate from a United States medical school, certain things seemed arguably true; for example, that women make just as good doctors as men. This, she wrote, is a true idea, and people will welcome it; it remains true for us today.

But other kinds of "true ideas" are more slippery. It used to be "true" that women needed several weeks in bed after childbirth. Then this was found to be actually harmful, so it became "true" that women should be moderately active as soon as possible after giving birth. Nowadays, it's "true" that birth is almost an outpatient procedure; most healthy mothers spend only a day or two in the hospital.

In obstetrics, as in the rest of medicine, "truth" is always a combination of economic necessity—in this case, the length of time a health insurance policy will cover—research results, fashion, and convenience. Each of us must discover for herself the truth of such ideas, and we need to trust our inner voices, not blindly accept the words of others.

THOUGHT FOR TODAY: I must learn to trust in my own judgment and keep true to my own beliefs.

Day 12

It is no matter whether I submit or rebel;
the event will still happen.

You neither know nor care for the truth of my heart;
but the truth of my body has all to do with you.
—JUDITH WRIGHT

Can the truth of the body be separated from the deepest wishes of the heart? If you are lucky, in pregnancy all the fragments of the self come together; you feel yourself a whole person. For some women, this may be the first experience of such wholeness, especially for a woman who has spent many years preparing herself for a profession, or working hard at a demanding job. The habit of thinking of yourself as a collection of separable entities—spirit, body, heart, brain—can be hard to shake.

Meditation soothes the spirit and quiets the anxiety that splits us off from ourselves. True, the process of life renewing itself will go forward whether any one individual submits or rebels; but you have chosen to participate in this process, and in surrendering to it you are fulfilling a vital part of your life's plan.

THOUGHT FOR TODAY: The truth of heart and body are one. I will surrender to the serenity of total congruence.

Day 13

*. . . as to the elves, having sought them in vain among
foxglove leaves and bells, under mushrooms and beneath the
ground-ivy mantling old wall-nooks, I had at length made up
my mind to the sad truth, that they were all gone out of
England to some savage country where the woods were wilder
and thicker, and the population more scant. . . .*

—CHARLOTTE BRONTË

Some of my earliest memories are of disappointments
similar to Charlotte Brontë's: the world of magic, which
seemed so close in fairy tales and nursery rhymes, must have
shut down just before I arrived on the scene. The haunted
houses were all gone, replaced by shopping malls. Movies put
some magic back into ordinary life, but the wonder was
missing.

The real magic years, of course, aren't a historical epoch
but a time in the life of every child. Having a baby gives you
a chance to revisit those years. You will spend time with a
little person who is thinking magically—who believes that
a beanstalk might grow up overnight, a frog might turn into a
prince, or a toy bought in a strange shop on Christmas Eve
might give birth to an army of creatures like itself.

Among the gifts of motherhood, recapturing your own
childhood isn't the first you think of; but it's a wonderful
surprise. These memories remind us of the richness of our
experience. We carry all our younger selves with us, wherever we go.

THOUGHT FOR TODAY: Motherhood gives me a chance to
share a second childhood before I've completely forgotten my
first.

> *A child is not a poem,*
> *a poem is not a child.*
> *There is no either/or.*
> *However.*
> —MARGARET ATWOOD

Women couldn't be/didn't need to be/didn't even want to be poets/artists/musicians, because they could have babies. This is the conventional wisdom our mothers grew up with; some of us grew up with it, too. But how strange it seems to think of pregnancy closing down options. Just the opposite is true: pregnancy expands your possibilities, opens the door to new experiences. Women can write poems, pilot planes, and govern countries in addition to having children.

You may want to put other possibilities on hold, though; bearing and rearing a child is so absorbing, physically and emotionally, that it doesn't leave much time and energy available for deeply creative work of other kinds. That's why parental leaves were invented. The more creative and demanding your work is, the more seriously you'll want to evaluate your readiness to return to it.

Babies don't substitute for other kinds of creativity; our creative powers are so great we can have them and write music, build buildings, or run offices, too. But we need to nurture ourselves to refresh our creativity.

THOUGHT FOR TODAY: Instead of either/or in my life, I'll think both/and—but maybe not all at the same time.

Day 15

I am a thief—and I am not ashamed. I steal from the best wherever it happens to be—

—MARTHA GRAHAM

Dancer and choreographer Martha Graham was talking about gestures and movements—how she watched people and used the way their bodies moved in her dances. But it might also be useful to be able to steal people's thoughts and feelings, to summon courage when you need it, or patience, or hope.

No doubt, people looking at you wish they could beg, borrow, or steal some of the nobility of your pregnancy. On days when you feel particularly tired or dumpy, remember that not only are you in a blessed condition, but your very existence is a symbol of hope for others. Can you steal back some of their admiration, some of the happiness they attribute to you?

We can't really steal thoughts, feelings, or movements from others, of course; what we can do is try to make them our own. And when we take an embracing gesture or a happy thought into our own bodies, it becomes an expression of our own possibility. Happiness is yours, for the borrowing.

THOUGHT FOR TODAY: I will practice the gestures and movements of enjoyment, and they will enhance my daily life.

Day 16

In the wilderness you are a spring.
You perpetually melt,
Lake and river maker, dedicated as the porpoise
To return to the sea.

—SANDRA McPHERSON

Some women experience pregnancy as a growing heat within their bodies; some have even compared it to light, "as though I had a lightbulb inside," one friend said. For her, the baby was a source of warmth and illumination, a comforting presence that she learned from constantly.

As you know by now, pregnancy raises the body temperature. In that sense, your baby is a source of heat. And when you pause for a moment to think of the many ways pregnancy connects you to life, to past and future, and to the world outside, you can see why it might be considered a source of enlightenment.

The increased blood supply that nourishes your baby can be seen by the eye. Your vagina and cervix are a beautiful, deep red, like a flower. Your breasts have grown larger and firmer, and the areolas of your nipples are also darker; they're becoming ready to feed your baby. Pregnancy nourishes and burnishes your body, as you nourish and sustain your baby.

THOUGHT FOR TODAY: Life is reflexive and self-renewing. Everything I give comes back to me.

Day 17

I read somewhere that pregnant women like to watch swimming turtles. Then I realized the connection between them and the child living inside of us who is also encased and slowly drifting in its own sea world, and I felt affirmed.

—AMY SHELDON

Everything that affirms your reality strengthens you in your connectedness to the sources of health and growth. Some pregnant women feel this strong connection right from the beginning, but for others it's more fragile and needs more affirmation. A trip to a zoo, an aquarium, Sea World, or even a pet shop can give you an image as powerful as swimming turtles.

Women whose work belongs to a world that seems remote from the simple, homely beauty of pregnancy and birth—factory workers or lawyers, for example—can come to feel estranged from their bodies and the grand process happening within. It's especially important for such women to find affirmations.

All women need to pay special attention during pregnancy to the substances with which they come in contact. Health care workers often recognize the possible hazards in their jobs from potent drugs or gases, but every pregnancy deserves an environment as free as possible from risks. Check out cleaning equipment, air filters, dyes or bleaches, solvents, and any other compound used where you work.

THOUGHT FOR TODAY: Your baby is a form of marine life right now, and it needs to be protected from pollutants.

Day 18

I dwell in Possibility—
A fairer house than Prose—
More numerous of Windows—
Superior—for Doors—
                        —EMILY DICKINSON

Right now your baby is dwelling in Possibility. All your thoughts about it are partly questions; numerous Windows shed light upon its future, and an infinite number of Doors are open to it.

At birth, these possibilities will both expand and contract. You will become acquainted with this being, who comes into the world with highly organized readiness for life but few techniques for expression. The great task for early parenting is to maintain the state of readiness, to guarantee that no doors or windows close before their time.

We all recognize that bringing up a child means making choices, and that every choice you make shuts out some others. But in the early months of your baby's life, while it learns its first momentous lessons, the maximum light and air are essential. Soon enough, some open doors must close; acquiring any skills involves training, and all training diminishes spontaneity. Babies' mouths can make beautiful liquid sounds until learning the sounds of a language shapes their muscles. We trust in the rightness of our decisions.

THOUGHT FOR TODAY: My notions of possibility will adjust to the reality of my baby's capacities.

Day 19

. . . there was nothing between her and the stars. The light was crystalline. There was no shimmer, no distortion through earth haze.

—Leslie Marmon Silko

There is nothing between you and your baby; you are one body. Any distorting "earth haze" comes from stereotypes or expectations. It would be a magnificent achievement if you could free yourself of assumptions and expectations and see your baby with absolute clarity as just what it is, no more and no less.

But hardly any relationships are wholly free of "earth haze"; all too often we see only what we're looking for. We share assumptions with our friends and relatives; they expect certain things from us, and we from them, and it's only human to have preconceived (no pun intended) notions about your baby as well.

Right now, the nurture you are supplying is pure; you don't need to make any decisions to care for your baby perfectly. This purity and simplicity will change when the baby is born, but if you are aware of the temptation to prejudge and classify you can overcome it. Your baby will be itself, casting its own light, and you'll have an undistorted view.

THOUGHT FOR TODAY: I will practice cultivating a "beginner's mind"—a way of seeing through the haze.

> *Seated*
> *like a foetus*
> *I look for*
> *the dream-seam*
>
> *What's inside?*
> *A sun?*
> —MAY SWENSON

All human beings carry a midline seam down our bodies, front and back; often hair grows along it, and in pregnancy its pigmentation sometimes darkens. The midline is an important location, because all our paired organs grow out from it— lungs, limbs, ovaries, eyes, ears, etc. Hair grows in a different direction on either side of the line.

What's inside your body's seam? A new human being; a new set of ears, eyes, and fingers to experience the world; a new brain and heart to imagine it afresh. You can hear your baby's heartbeat through a stethoscope now; it can hear your voice.

Your midline seam is a relic of embryological development: When the embryo is just a ball of cells, an organ called the notochord, which will develop into the spinal column, appears along a seam that divides the ball in two. The body's midline marks that early turning to a vertebrate form. You carry yours, as your child will carry her or his own.

THOUGHT FOR TODAY: My body is a living record of my history. Memories are preserved in my flesh, for me to use as I choose.

Day 21

Touch is the most basic, the most non-conceptual form of communication that we have. In touch there are no language barriers; anything that can walk, fly, creep, crawl, or swim already has it.

—INA MAY GASKIN

When we think of touch, we most often limit it to our hands, because they move according to our wishes, to stroke, poke, twist, or embrace. Yet our earliest experience of touch is much broader than the fingers' sensitive experience: the baby in the womb is touched all over by its mother's body, liquidly held and rocked by her heartbeat and her breath. Your baby knows what it is to be held long before your arms will hold it.

New parents are sometimes unsure of how to hold their baby; it is so precious, and seems so fragile. Mothers and fathers both fear that they'll harm it somehow. It's reassuring to think that long before you had the opportunity to handle your baby, you were touching and holding it, surely and well.

THOUGHT FOR TODAY: I'll remember that my body has the wisdom to do what my baby needs, even before I consciously think of it.

Day 22

I scarcely dared to look
to see what it was I was
I knew that nothing stranger
had ever happened, that nothing
stranger could ever happen.
—ELIZABETH BISHOP

Humans are such adaptable creatures that the marvelous becomes ordinary fairly soon. Perhaps at night, when you settle yourself for sleep, once in a while you think of the miracle going on inside you. Most of the time, you probably accept it as a matter of course.

Yet what could be more strange or more wonderful than becoming pregnant? Carrying a live child inside your body, preparing it for independent existence; preparing to nourish it physically and spiritually.

Perhaps it isn't really strange, as this process is certainly human. But it is wonderful, even if you don't maintain a constant state of wonder. The tiniest chemical details of what is happening to you are the most astonishing, if you think about it—flesh making new flesh, your body busily filtering, secreting, efficiently building up and breaking down organic compounds, with few or no signs of difficulty. If you choose it, you have a perpetual occasion for awe.

THOUGHT FOR TODAY: I'm grateful for the reminder that life is wonderful.

Day 23

Suddenly many movements are going on within me, many things are happening, there is an almost unbearable sense of sprouting, of bursting encasements, of moving kernels, expanding flesh.

—MERIDEL LeSUEUR

For many women, toward the end of the fifth month is when their pregnancies really "take off" and become evident. It's almost ironic that at a time when you may be feeling better than you ever have in your life, people around you first notice a change. It's less common these days to treat a pregnant woman like an invalid, but older people especially may act solicitous toward you, encouraging you to rest, to avoid exertion, to take it easy.

Yet by now you're an old hand at pregnancy; you know how much you can comfortably do. For many women, this is a deliciously sensuous time. Your appetite is good, your health is blooming; you may just have acquired some becoming new clothes. Maternity clothes used to be drab, but these days pregnant women can dare to be comfortable without sacrificing color or chic. You've got it, and you might as well flaunt it.

THOUGHT FOR TODAY: I can think of this as my flowering period, before my fruit ripens.

Day 24

The ocean spills upon the sands
Water with a thousand hands
And when the water all is spilled
The sands are dry, the ocean filled.
—SAMUEL HOFFENSTEIN

Most of the world's work is of this kind—repetitive, mechanical, needing to be done again every day, ceaselessly as the tides: cleaning, cooking, farming, bookkeeping, health care, legislative work, clerical work. Farmers can harvest crops as part of their work, but for most workers the palpable fruit of their labor is little, late, and very slow.

Pregnancy, on the other hand, results in the most important and delightful of products—a baby. Much of the work of pregnancy proceeds without your conscious effort, yet the result is something more wonderful than the most gifted artist can produce. You can anticipate greater fulfillment from this work than from any other you have ever done, and you deserve to be proud of yourself.

THOUGHT FOR TODAY: The world's rhythm of creation and destruction is working for me. I'm part of a great creative surge that produces great things.

Day 25

Women need to know that it is important to discuss child care with men before children are conceived or born. . . . Most women and men do not discuss the nature of child rearing before children are born because it is simply assumed that women will be caretakers.

—BELL HOOKS

A baby may appear to be a great reward for a minimum of work, but after it's born a huge amount of work suddenly needs to be done. The smoothest running household can be thrown into confusion by a new baby. There really is no way to plan for the disruption that a new baby brings; the best method is simply to accept what comes, to throw oneself open to the new necessities.

If the parents are truly partners, all tasks can be eased. Neither one need feel martyred by or excluded from child care. Only mother can feed the baby from her body, but her partner can certainly hold a bottle.

Often fathers feel some jealousy of the new baby. It absorbs the mother's attention as well as monopolizing her body in ways that can make it awkward for him to express affection. With all the attention a new baby demands, don't forget the father's changing needs, too.

THOUGHT FOR TODAY: All our patterns will shift; I will pray for the patience and sensitivity to meet them as they come.

> *Everywhere in the house*
> *is the need for order.*
> *The grandmother darns sheets*
> *before the children finish*
> *dreaming.*
> —ELIZABETH FOLLIN-JONES

Many pregnant women go through a phase called "nesting," when they have a lot of energy for domestic tasks associated with the coming of the baby. Painting walls, refinishing woodwork, knitting tiny garments, making curtains, or sanding furniture can absorb even women who have never enjoyed these activities before. We seem to need to order our surroundings in advance, as though we anticipate the disruption that will come with the new arrival.

Yield to your nesting impulses, even if they only lead you to the nearest department store. Your life won't have much order in the first six weeks or so of your baby's life; it's well to have things running as smoothly as possible beforehand.

Now is a good time to arrange for the help you'll need after the birth; ideally, someone should come in for at least a week or two to keep house and cook meals so that you can have as much time as you need to be with your baby. If this isn't possible, perhaps you can line up a series of friends and relatives who will help out for a day or half-day at a time.

THOUGHT FOR TODAY: Faith and hope comfort my spirit, but I'm going to need human help with meals and laundry.

Day 27

. . . my huge mother body . . . monthly sends a white-stone egg down from my natural mind, with the moon, each month, a possible life.

—KATE GREEN

Every month more or less during a woman's life there is a chance for a possible new life; four or five hundred chances over the course of a lifetime. Like the fact that we have extras of most of our vital organs—two kidneys, two lungs—this is an example of life's abundance. The rule seems to be *more than enough.*

A pregnant woman feels abundant. There's more of her than she needs, because she is more than herself; her "natural mind" or whatever name she gives to the force within her that secretes necessities and transforms energy into flesh is generous.

Generously, pregnancy prepares women's bodies for birth, and birth is a welcoming into the world, a hospitality to the new baby. Birth is not the first gesture of abundant welcome—the baby has been nourished, caressed, and protected for many months already—and it is certainly not the last. Yet it is one of the most striking. Once you have given birth, your body will feel hospitable whatever happens.

THOUGHT FOR TODAY: I'm grateful that life provides an abundant margin. I'll strive to be as generous toward those I love.

Day 28

The time has been full of a deep breath of content and waiting.
All good things lie in the future.

—REBECCA HARDING DAVIS

Some mornings the first thing you feel is the weird, tender blow of your baby's tiny fist or heel against your belly. If you can, let go of anxieties about the day's activities, work or study, relationships or family; breathe deeply and know that this is indeed the best time yet.

Such silent prayer—for conscious gratitude is prayer—comes easier with practice. Try to set aside a few moments every day to feel your health and happiness. Even in a difficult pregnancy, where the mother must take extraordinary care to protect herself and her baby, there is much occasion for gratitude. Be grateful for your doctor or midwife, and if you can't be grateful, think about finding a new birth attendant.

At this time of your life, you deserve to be surrounded by nurturing companions. Any influence in your life that roughens it should be examined to see if it can be smoothed.

THOUGHT FOR TODAY: I take deep breaths full of contentment and know good things lie in the future.

Day 29

Contraception, sixties activism, and feminism . . . changed the way women lived and thought about themselves.
—Francesca C. Fay & Kathy S. Smith

Nowhere is this more true than in pregnancy and childbirth. Feminist activists have changed the American way of birth totally, from an obstetrician's job to a partnership of women, their babies, and birth advisors.

Right now you are the most active person in this partnership. You nourish the new life and prepare for its future. Recent social changes have given women the opportunity to be equal partners in all their relationships, and these also have a spiritual significance, encouraging us to trust in ourselves and in our own sources of wisdom.

The most important lesson learned from any kind of activism is when to act and when to pass. You now can reap the advantages of generations of women struggling to think and act for themselves. They have given you choices about how to act, and when.

THOUGHT FOR TODAY: Rejoice in the knowledge that your baby has an active, choiceful mother.

Day 30

No one on earth ever had a greater chance for glory. The world to be won and nothing to be lost.

—ZORA NEALE HUSTON

All pregnant women can feel themselves full of glorious possibilities. And seizing this chance, you really aren't risking very much; the odds are overwhelmingly in your favor. Your world will be won, whatever happens, for your spiritual being is strengthened through your daily practice of prayer and meditation, and the personal growth you're experiencing will enrich the entire balance of your life.

A serene, well-nourished spirit is a noble achievement, and there is no better opportunity to attain one than now, while your body is home to a new life. Every birth brings a new world with it, and your perceptions are being heightened by your spiritual development.

The sense of expectant wonder can stay with you all your life; no gains need be lost. Even after your child has been born and grown, and is immersed in a separate life, these gifts can be yours to cherish forever.

THOUGHT FOR TODAY: The world is always mine to win, but this pregnancy sharpens my senses of gratitude and possibility.

Day 31

> . . . *Thou art the mother womb*
> *The one who creates mankind* . . .
> —BABYLONIAN MYTH

You and your baby are such a complete unit, and will be for a while after the birth, that even a well-adjusted father may feel somewhat left out. The whole process of pregnancy and birth, while it flowers from your relationship, also changes the relationship; it can interrupt intimacy, and the pleasures of parenting are new and different from the pleasures of being a couple.

Although most expectant fathers aren't conscious of it, many of them feel more than a little jealous of the new baby, the new life that claims your body and your spirit. This is perfectly normal. It's also normal for couples to experience a little friction in these months, sometimes powered by these unconscious feelings.

What should you do? Nothing, probably, except to let your partner know how precious your relationship is. Remind your partner and yourself that this new life is an expression of your commitment to one another. You too might be feeling a little forlorn; your partner's emotional focus seems to be on the baby rather than on you. We never stop needing emotional nurturance from those we love.

THOUGHT FOR TODAY: Birth can roughen the texture of a relationship. With patience and detachment, we can smooth it again.

THIS MONTH'S VISIT TO THE DOCTOR

Date:

Weight: Blood Pressure:

Weight Gain:

This Month's Signs of Pregnancy:

Changes in Eating:

Changes in Sleeping:

Changes in Activities/Energy Level:

Reflections:

Questions for Next Month's Visit:

Day 1

People overlap without our thinking about it. . . . It was possible for an ordinary Englishman to have seen both Elizabeth I and George I—in the flesh. . . . A person could have talked to Mr. Jefferson and seen a very young Ronald Reagan.

—CHARLES GOODRUM

What will your baby live to see? Maybe not queens or kings but almost certainly things you can't imagine. This child is a link in the chain, a witness to history, as well as an actor on the stage of world events.

You can help your child grow into a responsible actor— someone who thinks about consequences, who accepts responsibility for sharing the world with others. Now plastic bags foul our oceans; fertilizer runoff poisons our rivers; greed and fear push us toward violence of different kinds. Your baby's generation will need to create a new code of behavior to meet these and other circumstances.

Everything you do together, especially now, while the baby's still part of you, will have consequences for its later life. Talk to it gently and think of it with love and hope even when it kicks you or exhausts you. Your body makes a luxurious environment for these months when you are one, preparing your child to love and respect its surroundings, even though nothing in later life will ever be quite so warm and snug and totally gratifying.

THOUGHT FOR TODAY: Whatever future events it will witness, I am preparing my baby for creative action.

Day 2

My grandmothers are full of memories
Smelling of soap and onions and wet clay
With veins rolling roughly over quick hands. . . . .
—MARGARET WALKER

When you think of the old women in your family, do you imagine becoming like them? Almost certainly, your life differs from theirs, yet you'll grow old in time. We're very conscious of the ways time marks us: puberty, cyclical changes, the first gray hair, the first wrinkle. Our culture persuades us to despise the marks of age, and advertisers sell us products to delay or erase them.

Soon you'll have a new being to hold and to watch, a smooth-skinned, brand-new creature utterly unmarked by experience or memory. Your skin and hair and shape will go back to a nonpregnant state, but the other changes you've gone through will last longer. Though you can't see them, your mind and heart have been through as many changes as your body, maybe more; but spiritual changes are irreversible. And those are the experiences that mark the hands and faces of old women and make them beautiful.

THOUGHT FOR TODAY: Since there's nothing I can do about the marks of age, I will learn to see their beauty.

Day 3

The earth asks of us that we live through the winter with her if we seek to know her as she truly is.

—KAREN MALPEDE

Any process that lasts three-quarters of a year will have some winter to it, even in Florida or California—some down time, some days that are less than thrilling or gorgeous. There will be days that are just days, to be lived through as best you can. But you'll manage the lean times better if, like a frontier woman putting up tomatoes and peaches from her garden, you've preserved some of the fruits from your days of plenty.

When life seems golden and full of possibility, we automatically respond with good cheer and positive thinking; we can call on these feelings in days of more wintry emotional climate, too. Winter is necessary for our lives; we need some time for spiritual hibernation, drawing in our energies. But we need never be depressed.

We are all born with the ability to store up radiant energy. If you can bring welcome and acceptance to every phase of this pregnancy, you are treating yourself and your baby as well as possible. Ease is the goal, not constant excitement or pleasure, but the serenity that comes from a fulfilled heart.

THOUGHT FOR TODAY: My life is truly one of great blessings, winter and summer.

Day 4

There is no savor
more sweet, more salt

than to be glad to be
what, woman,

and who, myself,
I am . . .
  —DENISE LEVERTOV

Although we all know in a general way what elegant equipment the human body is, many women find it's in pregnancy that they really appreciate its intricate efficiency. And just because it is so intricate and usually functions so efficiently, there are dozens of opportunities for minor malfunctioning.

Some pregnant women develop varicose veins, dry skin, or other irritating symptoms. These inconveniences are related to the larger pattern of efficiency that assures the baby will be well cared for, supplied with a circulatory system, and nourished in chemically balanced fluids. Still, they're a great inconvenience to the mother. She may admire the body's wisdom in amplifying her blood supply and changing her chemical balance, yet still resent having to wear support stockings and use expensive lotions.

Your body is an exquisite machine, equipped with automatic controls and needing a minimum of repair. Your serenity will be enhanced when you can feel grateful for its complexity and its mostly smooth running.

THOUGHT FOR TODAY: The sweetness of gratitude can be tasted more fully when it alternates with a little salt, a little grit.

Day 5

When you have a healthy appetite there is no such thing as bad bread.

—GABRIEL GARCIA MARQUEZ

For many women, this mid-trimester is a happy time. Their appetites are healthy, their energy is high, and they revel in positive feelings. One woman asked her mother, "Why didn't you ever tell me having a baby was this much fun?" and her mother said, "You'd never believe me."

For others, it's not so much fun. Fatigue and discomfort get in the way. Even for women who were never picky eaters before, meals can come to seem like chores to be gotten through as quickly as possible. If this is true for you, let your nurse or doctor know. When it's difficult to eat the balanced diet your baby needs, more vitamin supplements may be prescribed.

Yet even discomfort can't wholly depress the high spirits of a pregnant woman. Today, congratulate yourself on your bravery. You deserve good feelings, for you are as courageous as any explorer journeying into the unknown.

THOUGHT FOR TODAY: Whether or not I enjoy being pregnant these days, I'll eat the best bread I can, with all the gusto I can manage.

Day 6

> *The earth is your mother,*
> *she holds you.*
> *The sky is your father,*
> *he protects you . . .*
> *We are together always.*
> *We are together always.*
> *There never was a time*
> *when this*
> *was not so.*
> —NAVAHO LULLABY

Not so long ago, pregnant women were discouraged from vigorous exercise. Some relatives may still look surprised or disapproving if you continue a strenuous fitness program, or begin one. But many women who never included aerobic exercise in their lives find pregnancy a good time to begin. Your local Y or community center offers activities tailored to your needs.

In-laws or grandparents may act shocked and ask, "What about the baby?" This is a good opportunity to reassure them; an accident could hurt you, but your baby is shielded from harm no matter what you do.

You can tell your relations that pregnant women have swum competitively, run marathons, ridden horses, and raced bicycles. A coordinated fitness program can be a gift to yourself. Active women often have an easier time of labor and delivery, in part because they're used to sustained effort. Everything you can do to enhance your health will reap dividends later on.

THOUGHT FOR TODAY: Another gift of pregnancy is the opportunity to care for my body in healthy new ways.

Day 7

Spores of bluefern growing in the hollows along the river bank float toward the water in silver-blue lines hard to see unless you are in or near them, lying right at the river's edge when the sun shots are low and drained. Often they are mistook for insects—but they are seeds in which the whole generation sleeps confident of a future.

—TONI MORRISON

Your possible future Nobel prize winner is nothing but a bulge at your midriff and a pattern of dots on a sonogram, but this child and its peers will make momentous decisions some day. How can you prepare it for the future? How can you ensure that whatever decisions are made will be life-affirming ones?

You can't, of course. All you can do is your best, here and now. But if your child grows up in a home where love and understanding are abundant, then success is assured. A child's needs include the need for firm limits, for children learn self-discipline from being with disciplined adults.

Cleanse your mind and heart of unproductive worry. There is so much bad news every day that it's easy to let it dim your vision of the future. Prophets are scarce, though messengers of bad news seem to be plentiful; remind yourself that neither you nor anyone else can predict the future and keep your focus on the present, where the action is.

THOUGHT FOR TODAY: I can't see it or control it, but the things I do here and now will affect the future. Unconditional love is the best protection I can give my child for whatever lies ahead.

Day 8

Instead of saying that every woman is the Superior Woman *when she makes the right choices, why not trust that each woman has her own answers within her and her own individual timing?*

—BONNIE FISHER

In the days of family doctors, it wasn't uncommon for the same doctor to care for several generations of women in the same family. But no daughter had the same experience as her mother, nor will you; every woman, every baby, is different from every other. We each have our own rhythms, our own patterns of muscular development, holding on and letting go. No one can know in advance exactly what your birthing experience will be; all they—and you—can do is your best.

Pregnancy can be a puzzle for a first-time mother. You don't know whether to hang loose or come on strong, assert yourself or let things take their course. There seem to be no patterns to follow. Relax and have faith that what you are doing is right for you. If it isn't, you won't feel good about it. If you don't feel good about it, you have the opportunity to change it.

THOUGHT FOR TODAY: The only power I have is power over my own actions, but I have the right to surround myself with congenial spirits.

Let the pure sky ahead, this sky of long
and sweeping clouds, send to me
a wind so strong, a wind the scent of joy;
let all be born now, cleansed of dreams.
                                    —SIMONE WEIL

Most pregnant women have vivid, anxious dreams, sometimes grotesque or frightening, about birth. If you've never had a baby before, or seen a woman give birth, it is something of a mystery; fantasies can tap your childhood fears and serve them up freshly in your dreams. It's very common to dream that your baby is monstrous in some way, an alien or fantastic creature, strangely deformed or powerful. These dreams are a way of handling normal anxieties; they have no meaning beyond your own mental state.

It's also normal to have high expectations for your child. Successful parents want successful children; young mothers often brag about how early their babies smile, roll over, walk, or talk, as though they could take credit for these achievements. But if you reach down deeply within you, you know that your child is another person, soon to be outside you. Credit for children's success belongs to them, not to their parents.

THOUGHT FOR TODAY: Purity and joy belong to everyone, and they flow more easily where neither fears nor expectations are laid. What will be, will be; I'm responsible only for my part.

Day 10

I have observed that generally women take more pleasure when they are with child than when they are not with child, not only in eating more and feeding more luxuriously, but taking a pride in their great bellies, although it be a natural effect of a natural cause.

—Margaret Cavendish, Duchess of Newcastle

How do you feel about your "great belly"? Are you sometimes definitely proud, wearing it like a badge of honor, and sometimes ashamed because it seems a sign of weakness? Many pregnant women feel both stronger and more vulnerable; their feelings vacillate between pride and humiliation.

But at this time most women take a lot of pleasure in the ordinary physical details of life. Often your skin and hair feel especially sleek and healthy, because you're taking such good care of yourself, eating well, sleeping a lot, exercising. You may have noticed some changes in the pigmentation of your skin; the central line of the body often becomes darker, patches of darker coloring appear on the face. These signs will probably go away after the birth, but your health and pleasure can continue as long as you want.

THOUGHT FOR TODAY: The great belly is a badge of honor, and the good health habits it has brought me can be lifelong.

Day 11

What you say of the pride of giving life to an immortal soul is
very fine, dear, but I cannot enter into that; I think much
more of our being like a cow or a dog at such moments; when
our poor nature becomes so very animal and unecstatic. . . .
—QUEEN VICTORIA

Poor Queen Victoria! From this excerpt of a letter to one
of her daughters, it doesn't sound as though she had much
pleasure or pride from her many pregnancies.

You are in a position to enjoy every possible moment of
your pregnancy, unconstrained by false modesty. You can
have the pride of giving life to an immortal soul *and* the
shameless joy of feeling good inside your skin. Massaging your
nipples to get them ready for nursing should give you
pleasure, and so should your daily exercise routine. Kinship
with your true nature can be a source of learning for you, not
shame.

Many women find their senses heightened during pregnancy; sometimes this sensitivity can bring discomfort, such
as sudden nausea at the smell of gasoline or carbon monoxide,
but it can also give daily life a special radiance. The colors of
fruits and vegetables in a market; the sounds of music; the
touch of soft fabrics or your partner's skin; all are keen
pleasures, little sources of ecstasy.

THOUGHT FOR TODAY: For me, there need be no conflict
between physical pleasure and spiritual ecstasy. My well-
being is what's important.

Day 12

> *then the earth itself*
> *will turn and turn and cry out*   *oh I*
> *have been made sick*
>
>   *then you*   *my little bud*
>   *must flower and save it*
>   —GRACE PALEY

It is normal to feel an occasional pang of despair at the state of the world your baby's coming into, even guilt because our generation hasn't cared better for it. You know you aren't responsible for industrial pollution, nuclear radiation, or the exploding national debt. Yet sometimes it seems like a shabby sort of world to hand down.

All our children will have spiritual paths of their own to travel, and their own way of coping with the world's imperfections. If life in your household is environmentally conscious, it will include global thinking and a sense of personal responsibility toward the environment. No one knows how the future of our planet will develop. Our individual lives are only a tiny piece of a pattern vaster than we can imagine, and if we trust that the pattern has its own wisdom and obeys its own laws, we can be serene in the knowledge that we're doing the best we can.

THOUGHT FOR TODAY: Saving the world is too big a task for me or my baby, but we can live gently in it, with gratitude for its gifts.

Day 13

What life was there, was mine

now and again to lay
one hand on a warm brick

and touch the sun's ghost
with economical joy

now and again to name
over the bare necessities.
—ADRIENNE RICH

Your baby's sense organs are all formed now. You may have noticed how its movements respond to music; it has eyelids and complete fingernails, and sensory receptors have developed in the skin. The rest of its growth will be fat and muscle tissue; the basic equipment is all in place.

Life gives each one of us much more than the bare necessities. Our bodies are lavishly furnished with alternate pathways, fail-safe mechanisms, and backup plans. If we economize on our feelings, it's our own decision to do so. Love and joy are infinitely renewable resources: the more we spend, the more we get. Practice now removing conditions from the love you give. Life itself directs us toward abundance and generosity.

THOUGHT FOR TODAY: I'll put no restraints on the love I show my baby. I am capable of infinite patience and generosity and have faith that my powers of loving and giving will be equal to the demands placed on them.

Day 14

If you're strong, you know that life's a road on which you're always alone, even with love, even if people have halted along the way to engage your emotions.

—MONIQUE PROULX

Literally a pregnant woman cannot be alone; she carries in her body a child who symbolizes her commitment to a partner and to a family. Some women who enjoy solitude find that pregnancy crowds them. A friend told me about waking one morning while she was carrying her third child to find her bed occupied not just by her own pregnant body and her husband, but both their young children, two cats, and the family dog. All slept peacefully except her; she had been pushed against the wall.

To find serenity at such a time, you must go deep within yourself, to the still place in your spirit where you are most yourself though never alone. Even when you feel lonely, you are accompanied; our companion on life's journey is a power greater than our understanding, a spiritual guide that acts always in our best interest.

THOUGHT FOR TODAY: From time to time I need to seek refuge; yet though I may welcome solitude, I am never alone.

> *what is it like to have*
> *a child afraid of you, your own*
> *child, your first child, the one*
> *who must forgive you if either of you are to*
> *survive . . . ?*
>
> —ALTA

There's probably no way you can avoid conflict with your child after it's born and active in the world. The early months are almost like a honeymoon, if you and the baby find a good rhythm of sleeping, feeding, waking, and playing. But if you don't—if your baby seems to be a confirmed night owl and a sound daytime sleeper, or an every-hour feeder, or has colic or some other distress—then you may encounter conflict early.

New parents often judge themselves harshly if they find the stark realities of life with baby more than they can bear serenely. Be as gentle with yourself as you'd like to be with your child. You're doing your best. Don't expect yourself to have superhuman energy and forbearance. Remember that your baby isn't capable of malice or manipulation; she or he is obeying simple laws of survival.

Prayer and meditation will help keep you on an even keel. All parents make mistakes, but with spiritual guidance you can avoid doing anything your child will have to forgive later.

THOUGHT FOR TODAY: I can't control my feelings, but I can control my actions. And I can nurture the child within me, too.

Day 16

". . . where does one read a deeper tale than upon the most perfectly printed page of the most precious book? Upon the blank page."

—Isak Dinesen

Everyone who's ever observed newborn babies understands that they're not "blank pages"; they come into the world with a small set of behavioral responses like sucking, cooing, crying, and blinking, and they are sensitive to what their parents expect from them. They also have an enormous capacity for learning.

Very early, within the first two years, they learn femininity or masculinity. Little girls learn to act "feminine"— concerned with their appearance—from being expected to act that way. Little boys are boisterous, adventurous, and curious because their parents expect them to be that way from birth. Babies are skilled at picking up cues, and within their individual set of potential behaviors they learn very fast what their parents consider appropriate.

If you expect a little girl to be active and curious, she will be, just as little boys will be tender and domestic if they're encouraged in that direction. Bear in mind that their little pages aren't blank, although some of the writing may temporarily be invisible.

THOUGHT FOR TODAY: I will do my best to spare my child useless stereotyping, and to evoke the potential for as full a life as possible.

Day 17

. . . clinging to the habits of the past gives all of us some comfort in this thus-far-unexplained universe: it is always reassuring to think that our ancestors "did it" the same way.
—LORRAINE HANSBERRY

Female friends and relatives are eager to share how they "did it," aren't they? It's amazing how a pregnant woman evokes intimate narratives from people who are normally quite reserved, tales of screams and laughter and blaring sirens. Many women become proselytizers for certain techniques or details: "I had one baby with Lamaze and one without, and *let me tell you* . . ." Yet every woman delivers her babies in her own unique way. Other women's stories are interesting and moving, but they probably don't have much relevance for you.

Remember that no matter what you expect, the power is out of your hands. Surrender your worries and doubts, your grandiose expectations and your fears; the power that will direct the birth of your child belongs to all humanity, not just to your family. Have faith in the rightness of your life, and all will be well.

THOUGHT FOR TODAY: My baby and I are part of a greater whole—an essential part, but only a part.

Day 18

Giving her perishable
souvenir of hope, a dull
white outside and smooth-
edged inner surface
glossy as the sea, the watchful
maker of it guards it
day and night . . .
—MARIANNE MOORE

Your abdomen bears an egg-shaped oval swelling, your "souvenir of hope," and the watchful maker also guards it, though it's a good deal more secure than the sea bird's egg described in the poem. You don't have to think about your child's welfare because it's so well cared for, day and night.

During this month many women find their sleep interrupted, even if they haven't experienced this before. Often a woman will wake to urinate, or she'll have a vivid dream that begs to be written down, or a particularly vigorous fetal movement will jar her awake. It's almost as though she were being trained to sleep more lightly, to sleep with one eye open and one ear cocked. For some mothers these months are useful training.

Some women are naturally light sleepers, of course, and some don't experience wakefulness at this point in their pregnancies. All babies are different, and their patterns of sleep and waking will be worked out in the early weeks. They'll still be watched over day and night—and so will you.

THOUGHT FOR TODAY: My spiritual welfare is safeguarded as carefully as my baby's physical well-being.

Day 19

. . . it was only when I had children of my own to appreciate and to study that I finally realized the full extent of the distance I had traveled.

—PETER USTINOV

Someone has said that the real miracle of family life is not that adults make children but that children make adults. Some people dread becoming parents for this reason—it means a kind of death to them, an end of youth and a giving up of youthful hopes.

It's quite usual even for people who are eager to have children to share fears like these. Becoming parents, for most of us, carries a heavy subconscious meaning: becoming like *our* parents, who were the staid, serious guardians of our youth. Or perhaps they were irresponsible or abusive, figures that inspired us with fear and pity.

You needn't be afraid that you are destined to repeat any aspects of your parents' behavior that you don't want for yourself and your family. You have the power to choose what kind of parent you will be. You can measure the distance you travel however you like.

THOUGHT FOR TODAY: Joy and sadness don't belong to either youth or adulthood, but to life. My parenting can be as young or old as I choose.

My belly has tracks on it—
*   hands and feet*
are moving
under this taut skin.
In snow, in light,
we are about to become!
—KATHLEEN FRASER

Your body is your child's landscape, its entire world. Women sometimes feel uneasy at this enormous responsibility; if this is your case, remember that we're not called on to give more than we have. A power greater than your individual spirit is directing your destiny and your child's, and all will be well.

When you calm your fears, you can feel a strong connection to this higher power. Your child's unborn spirit connects with it, too. Your lives are one life now, twinned and woven together. Soon you'll be two separate lives, though your connection is lifelong. But your mutual connection to a source of spiritual guidance is stronger than the bond between you, and you can safely turn your common welfare over to it. Your baby will have the protection it needs even after it leaves your womb.

THOUGHT FOR TODAY: My baby's world will change even faster than mine. I'm grateful for the higher power that protects us both.

Day 21

It was the twenty-sixth week when this happened . . . I was very, very upset. The part about remaining flat on my back didn't sink in for about a day. Then suddenly I said, "Flat on my back! I can't even go to the office?" They said, "No, you don't understand. You don't go anywhere!"

—JANE METZROTH

There is a condition that medical people call, perhaps unkindly, "incompetent cervix"—it means the muscles of the cervix aren't strong enough to hold the uterus closed against the pressure of the growing baby. Women who have this are usually ordered to stay in bed for several months, and sometimes doctors tighten the cervix surgically, as well.

A woman who has this complication might want to struggle hard against that word "incompetent." She's pregnant in the best way she can be, right now, whatever happens, and it's foolish to try to compare her with others, to compete for perfection. The glory of humankind is our diversity; each cervix is different; each family is different; each baby will be different.

Thinking in averages, in statistics, is a shortcut, an oversimplification. It's important that you appreciate your full measure of individual complexity, taking each day as it comes. You've never traveled this road before; be assured that whatever you meet will welcome you, even if it appears forbidding.

THOUGHT FOR TODAY: Like the courageous Jane Metzroth, my spirit is equal to what I must do.

Day 22

I am for keeping the thing going while things are stirring;
because if we wait till it is still, it will take a great while to get
it going again.

—SOJOURNER TRUTH

Events have a momentum of their own, as Sojourner
Truth knew, and often the wisest course is to surrender
ourselves to it. No two pregnancies are exactly alike, nor are
any two births; they may correspond to roughly the same
pattern, but every mother and baby are an individual pair.

The action of your hormones during pregnancy is something like stirring; after the first few months, your metabolism
increases steadily until birth. Most women feel warmer than
usual during pregnancy; for someone whose fingers and toes
are often chilly, this can be a pleasure. And your blood volume
increases by almost half again. These progesterone-induced
changes are often accompanied by emotional turbulence,
perhaps alternating with great tranquillity.

Being stirred needn't upset you. Give yourself to the
rapid changes that are happening in your body and spirit—
you are stronger than you know.

THOUGHT FOR TODAY: My tranquil spirit can survive
turbulence, even welcome it.

Day 23

The trees (are) luxurious. . . . They know if it isn't raining now it soon will. One needn't worry; it is O.K. to spread one's crown as beautifully as one can.

—CAROL BLY

For some women, pregnancy is the first time in their lives that they feel like spreading their crowns, luxuriating in their physicalness. Partly this may be a feeling of release from cultural images of extreme thinness; no one can expect a pregnant woman, doing the world's most important work, to look like a bathing-suit model. Give yourself permission to be the size you are.

If you do feel liberated, perhaps you can find ways to hold on to this positive self-image after your baby comes. Feeling beautiful and sexy is a gift; it can be with you always, as long as you're healthy. You don't need cultural stereotypes or the admiration of others to support you; your radiance will speak for itself.

THOUGHT FOR TODAY: Pregnancy, birth, nursing, and mothering are all beautiful activities—just participating in them makes me beautiful.

Day 24

I think that my soul is red
like the soul of a sword or a scarlet flower . . .
—CHARLOTTE MEW

Red, color of blood, has many meanings in different cultures. Most women aren't distressed by the sight of blood; it's familiar to us from our menstrual fluid. Men may be disturbed by blood, which they associate only with injury, but we know it's also a sign of healthy life. In Chinese tradition, it's a bridal color; in Christian iconography it's associated with sin but also with sacrifice; in Indian art red is the color of creation and destruction.

Scientific opinion is still divided about whether babies can actually see inside the womb; if they can, what they see is red, the vivid, vital red of mother's blood. What's certain is that newborn babies respond to brilliant primary colors, especially red.

The world your baby inhabits is a brilliant red now, because of the increased blood supply that nourishes your pregnancy. If you have any lingering squeamishness about the sight or thought of blood, now is a good time to work on getting rid of it. Blood is beautiful; it's the fluid of life.

THOUGHT FOR TODAY: My body is miraculous; nothing about it is ugly or shameful.

Day 25

There are some people who cannot get onto a train without imagining that they are about to voyage into the significant unknown; as though the notion of movement were inseparably connected with the notion of discovery, as though each displacement of the body were a displacement of the soul.

—MARGARET DRABBLE

Movements of the body are movements of the soul, for we are unified creatures; there are no wounds or caresses that don't affect both body and spirit. You aren't pregnant simply in your body; your spirit is also preparing for motherhood, growing along with your baby until the day of birth brings you face to face.

Not only movement but also time is connected with discovery. When we have a secret, we know in time it will be made known. Human growth is such a secret, like the unfolding of a bud; the form of life exists potentially long before it can be felt, seen, or heard.

Each step in the growth of the body is also a spiritual step. For every stage in our development there are corresponding discoveries; even developments that may seem like negatives—such as the restricted movements of late pregnancy, or the gnarls and wrinkles of age—can bring us to new thresholds of consciousness, of gratitude, if we approach them in a positive frame of mind.

THOUGHT FOR TODAY: I can be a traveler who greets each stage on my journey with gladness and gratitude.

> *The mind*
> *reflects*
> *the happiness*
> *of the body*
> *and echoes*
> *its old pains*
> *as wild grapes*
> *stain*
> *the leaves that*
> *arch around*
> *them*
> —MARTY ROTH

Our feelings live in our bodies as well as in our minds; our muscles hold old fears and humiliations longer, sometimes, than our minds remember them. If you are carrying anxieties around with you, now is a good time to learn to let them go.

First you need to recognize that you are holding onto old tensions; then you may need help to release them. A good massage therapist can help you relinquish old patterns that keep pain and fatigue in your body instead of ease and pleasure.

Now, of all times, you should be good to yourself. You need vitality to carry and bring forth your child. If past sadness and fear are keeping your muscles tense or sore, then energy isn't flowing through your body as freely as it could. You owe yourself liberation from past pain.

THOUGHT FOR TODAY: If I am carrying old anxieties with me, I learned how to keep them; I can learn to let them go.

Day 27

Strange how a patch of muddy shore

in the light would seem, if we stopped,
to hold the key to what we've always known,
desired: water, solitude, a story
we've come from that's waiting to resume.
— ALISON CLARK

If you have another child, this pregnancy may seem very much like a story you've "come from that's waiting to resume"—the visits to your doctor or midwife, the vitamins you take, even the clothes you wear are vivid reminders of something you've already known. But this baby will have its unique story to tell, beginning with its birth.

Of course, every birth changes a family's configuration. You become parents for the first time, or your only child acquires—and becomes—a sibling. Even in large families, where you'd think one more or less wouldn't matter, a new baby introduces a new personality and changes every relationship in the family.

The story of our families' lives is written freshly every moment. We hold the key to success when we let go of expectations and practice wonder and acceptance.

THOUGHT FOR TODAY: I will welcome my new baby on its own terms, without making assumptions.

Day 28

To wake at three
and read the ceiling
is more than a smear
of the infinite
—GEOFF PAGE

During a monthly visit, a woman nearing the end of her second trimester complained to her obstetrician that she woke up at night. "Every night, almost exactly the same time," she said. "Three o'clock! The house is cold, and I don't want to wake my husband, so I just lie there. What can I do?"

"Get up," he told her. "Do your housework. Do office work. Do something, but use the time."

The next night, sure enough, she woke. She found it was difficult to make herself get out of bed, but once she was up and wrapped in a woolly robe, she could pay bills, do laundry, even get through work she'd brought home from the office.

Over the next week, in fact, she found that without the usual daytime interruptions she could get through a great deal of office work in the middle of the night, so that when she got drowsy after a couple of hours she didn't mind sleeping in and coming to work late. Not everyone can be quite so flexible, perhaps, but you can use those wakeful small hours for something more productive than contemplating infinity.

THOUGHT FOR TODAY: My time is too precious to squander. If I get a dividend in the middle of the night, I'll use it constructively.

Day 29

I always build a house when I start something new in my life.
That's my custom. I'm like a snail crawling along with a shell
on its back. I build a house, and then I start roaming around.
—CHIYO UNO

Human beings need a secure base from which to start.
It's built into our biology, unlike fish or insects, which develop
rapidly, sometimes in constant motion; we mammals need to
go through a relatively long period of secure housing before
we're called on to start roaming around.

Your baby's house is the fluid-filled amniotic sac inside
your uterus, built by the two of you out of the finest
materials—your own cherished body. This home provides a
period of security from which your baby will launch into the
cool brightness of a world of infinite possibility.

All our lives, humans reach for some version of the
warmth and flexibility of the womb. Many of us, if we're
lucky, find it in our intimate relationships. The nourishment
we get prepares us to meet whatever challenge greets us.

THOUGHT FOR TODAY: The real home I seek is shelter for
my spirit. With this foundation, I can grow in any direction.

Day 30

The insects walk over our warm skin.
They think we are the earth.
                                        —LINDA HOGAN

The still, flat surface of beds and tables must be terribly strange to newborn babies, who are accustomed to a soft liquid world of curves and caresses. Life outside is hard and cold; it's for this reason that in many cultures new babies are carried for a time close to someone's skin—the mother's, perhaps, or an older sibling's.

These days we also see new fathers carrying their babies in slings or pouches, a good way to reassure your child and accustom it gradually to the world. When your infant can hear the reassuring bass note of a heartbeat (even though it's outside, not inside, the body), smell familiar breath, and feel the warmth of skin, it's less likely to be fussy and mistrustful.

Modern life does not allow most new parents to carry their babies with them constantly, but it's a good idea to invest in a well-made baby carrier of some sort for those times when you can. Very soon your body will cease to be the whole world to your baby, but your closeness can give it warmth and reassure it that the new world is a place to be happy.

THOUGHT FOR TODAY: I want easy transitions for my baby; there will be enough difficulties in life without our creating them.

Day 31

There is no way we can meet the day with a strong enough sense of the holy.

—LYNN STRONGIN

Today is roughly the end of your second trimester. By now you've seen that medical schedules for human pregnancy are still rather sketchy; you may have noted that your development follows its own path, regardless of what the books say.

You may believe you want to know in advance the exact details of your baby's birth, its sex (if you don't already know it), its size, its mode of arrival, its temperament. But this desire is really an expression of your anxiety, a seeking to control the uncontrollable. Your baby will be who it is, and advance warning can't really ease your relationship.

Each of the millions of women who are pregnant on the planet right now has her own individual timetable, and each in her own way is surrendering to the mysteries of growth. For every one of you, the day brings with it a special realization of the holiness of life. Even if you don't leap up in the morning with a praise song on your lips, you can greet the world with glad prayers in your own style.

THOUGHT FOR TODAY: I don't need advance planning to be the best mother I can be. What I need is to surrender my spirit to a greater power.

THIS MONTH'S VISIT TO THE DOCTOR

Date:

Weight: Blood Pressure:

Weight Gain:

This Month's Signs of Pregnancy:

Changes in Eating:

Changes in Sleeping:

Changes in Activities/Energy Level:

Reflections:

Questions for Next Month's Visit:

Day 1

> *i am the goddess*
> *and it is my blood*
> *that you ride to freedom*
> *i am the goddess*
> —GERRY MELOT

When you feel your baby moving these days, you can feel the power of the universe streaming through you. Your body is a world and you and your baby are its peoples. For many women, these feelings of power are new and strange; lifelong habits of gentleness and humility make it hard to acknowledge the immense power of creation that resides within.

Your goddess-self is the part of you that feels at one with the universe, the part of your body and spirit that blossoms into kinship with all creation. In this trimester you can get used to your power, for you'll need it when the baby comes. All at once, you and your partner will be faced with the management of another human being, one who will grow from utter dependence to independence, struggling every step of the way. You'll need strength. If all people could use their power creatively, as you're doing now, our world would reflect those values.

THOUGHT FOR TODAY: I long for a world in which all people can tap the divinity that lives within them.

Day 2

> *But there are hours of lonely musing,*
> *Such as in evening silence come,*
> *When, soft as birds their pinions closing,*
> *The heart's best feelings gather home.*
> —CHARLOTTE BRONTË

When the bustle of the day is over and you have some quiet time with your baby, then the heart's best feelings can gather. The love you feel for your baby and for your whole future family can strengthen you, so that you are both eager to know your family's future and patient enough to wait for it serenely.

Your baby can hear drumbeats; have you noticed a change in its movements when you listen to strongly rhythmic music? If you read poetry aloud, perhaps it can sense the rhythm in the words. When your thoughts soar, perhaps they flood it with happiness.

The spiritual bond between you and your baby is soft and strong as a bird's wing. It can lift your thoughts to a high plane and fold them in to peaceful contemplation. The strength may have something to do with your baby's bones growing longer and stronger—you need lots of calcium and magnesium now, to help its frame develop. But the softness is in your heart, full of love and eager for goodness.

THOUGHT FOR TODAY: I can gather both strength and softness in whatever solitude I can find.

Day 3

> *When light unfolds*
> *it assumes the shape*
> *of what the eye*
> *is inventing*
> —JOSE EMILIO PACHECO

You know your baby so well, yet you don't know him or her at all. Your thoughts about the future are wishes and fears that belong to you, not really to the baby. It will have its own mind and spirit, and will lead its own life. Your baby may not want what you want, nor choose what you would choose for it.

Sometimes you may find yourself predicting the new direction your family will take, thinking you know what life will be like after this baby's birth. Remember how frustrated you felt when you were a child, and grown-ups in your family thought they understood what you were thinking or feeling? All you really know is that you don't know how this birth will affect your family. Your baby will surprise you, and you'll all grow together.

THOUGHT FOR TODAY: I will work at the practice of detachment so that I can avoid the danger of seeing only what my eyes want to see.

Day 4

. . . buried amid the discomforts and disgust was an untrammeled delight, the nature of which I wouldn't fashion into words, but which was wholly enviable.

—ROBERTA ISRAELOFF

Your baby can see light through the skin of your abdomen, through the layers of fat and the fluids surrounding it. That means it can also perceive darkness—although nighttime doesn't discourage most babies from moving around. The most comfortable position for you in bed is usually lying on your side, with one leg slightly raised, so that your whole belly rests next to you and the baby's gestures are less disturbing.

Remember how eagerly you waited for the first sign of movement? There are times now when you probably wish wholeheartedly that your baby would slow down, or even stop moving—because you know that can be one sign of readiness for birth.

When you let yourself float with the baby, you can see how futile those eagernesses or regrets are. There is no hurrying this process. It's growing in its own time, as you are changing in yours.

THOUGHT FOR TODAY: I am learning to accept that everything that happens to us is as it should be.

Day 5

. . . I felt sure that it had been my past that helped make the future possible. The women in my family had acted as if their lives were meaningful. Their lives were art.

—JEWELLE GOMEZ

Has this pregnancy brought you closer to the women in your family? You may not have had particularly intimate relationships with your mother, your grandmothers, or your aunts and great-aunts, yet many women find they feel very connected to their female relations in late pregnancy, and they want to hear stories about the births of all the children in the family.

You're lucky if you come from a family where storytelling is an art, especially if you are close to your mother and grandmothers. No matter what else happens to a woman, whether she's a factory worker or a federal judge, the births of her children are deeply meaningful events in her life, and they deserve to be celebrated.

Families should preserve women's stories of pregnancy and birth, so that children can have a sense of the tradition from which they come. If your baby is a girl, she may carry that tradition on when she has children of her own. It's dizzying to think right now of future generations, but this is how the past prepares the future.

THOUGHT FOR TODAY: My baby's birth will link me to my own past as well as to the future.

Day 6

These are her endless years, woman and child, in dream
molded and wet, a bowl growing on a wheel,
not mud, not bowl, not clay, but this becoming,
winter and split of darkness, years of wish.
—MURIEL RUKEYSER

Here you are on the homestretch, growing larger almost daily, immersed in preparing for your baby's entrance into the world. Have you neglected yourself, in attending to this important Other? It wouldn't be surprising if you have begun to cut corners in your daily rituals of self-care and of spiritual practice. Between your work, your home, your relationships, and your pregnancy, *you* are in danger of being squeezed out. It may feel perfectly all right to neglect your spiritual needs: "Everything's fine," you may feel. "I can go on automatic pilot for a while." But you may find, as a friend of mine says, that pretty soon you're running on fumes.

Our spiritual center needs regular replenishment. You're too important to neglect; regular prayer and meditation will nourish your spirit, and you'll find that every aspect of your life will repay this deliberate effort. Pregnancy can be such a fulfilling experience. It would be a shame to let fatigue rob you of its possibilities.

THOUGHT FOR TODAY: I am the most important person in my life and, for a little while longer, in my baby's. I deserve to treat myself accordingly.

Day 7

The lore of motherhood is a science which is now beginning, but it is not following the lines which convention and the moralists expect. It defies sentiment, ridicules unnecessary and unintelligent sacrifice, and is not content to suffer, but makes demands.

—DORA RUSSELL

Nowadays we understand that what is best for the mother is almost always best for the baby; that there is no particular virtue in sacrifice or suffering; and that women by and large are experts on their own female anatomy and biology. But it's well to bear in mind that this was not always the case, and that our foremothers' victories didn't come easily.

Much in our system of medical care still needs changing, especially obstetrical care, although the range of choices available to many mothers is now wonderfully wide. Sophisticated medical technology should be deployed only for the benefit of mothers, and they should decide when and whether to use it.

Since you are going to be in charge of your own care, you need a strong sense of your own right to make decisions. Reflection will enable you to tell the difference between what you can change and what you must accept, and to know when you need to ask for help.

THOUGHT FOR TODAY: I'm the central character in the drama of my life, and I deserve truly supporting players.

Day 8

Seeing you brave and water-clean,
Leaven for the heavy ones of earth,
I am swift to feel that what makes
The plodder glad is good . . .
—ANNE SPENCER

Babies are a leaven for all heaviness. Some behavioral scientists believe there's a scientific basis for the delight they bring, that the particular shape of a baby's head and eyes is uniquely able to evoke protective warmth from adults. It's true that the sourest pessimist will smile at a baby.

The perfection of detail in a baby's body is a source of great gladness to parents: the narrow fold of eyelid, tiny lashes, translucent fingernails more delicate than seashells, miniature fingers, toes, and ears. In these finely sculpted features we see more clearly than in our own bodies the miraculous care with which we've been created.

The magical freshness lasts only a short time, the fleeting childhood years, but the miracle remains. This work of love you carry within you is the finest product of human creativity, and it will spread gladness throughout your world.

THOUGHT FOR TODAY: Babies refresh our souls by reminding us of the infinite artistry of our creator.

Day 9

*. . . sharing joy is absolutely superior . . . to sharing suf-
fering. Gladness, not sadness, is talkative, and truly human
dialogue differs from mere talk or even discussion in that it is
entirely permeated by pleasure in the other person and what
he says. It is tuned to the key of gladness, we might say. . . .*
— HANNAH ARENDT

Everyone needs intimate friends. Sharing joy doubles it,
so they say, while sharing sorrow halves it. And though
pregnancy is a time of joy for the most part, most pregnant
women have occasional fears or sadnesses; confiding them to
a sympathetic listener diminishes their power to color your
outlook.

Many women find friends through groups or classes
organized by birth advisors—obstetricians, midwives, or hospitals. Your husband or partner may be your best friend, but
another pregnant woman can bring special understanding to
both your anxieties and your satisfactions.

That is one excellent reason for you to attend childbirth
or labor classes, and besides, you'll learn useful information
about the birth process. No one can guarantee you a swift
delivery, but women who have taken care to educate themselves about labor and delivery almost always have a more
pleasant time. And the friends you make in such groups or
classes can be with you—and your baby—for years.

THOUGHT FOR TODAY: My bonds with others are a source
of companionship and support in my progress toward birth.

Day 10

The voice of the sea speaks to the soul. The touch of the sea is sensuous, enfolding the body in its soft, close embrace.

—KATE CHOPIN

The rhythm of the sea persists independently of any human effort. To walk along the seashore, or to play in the surf at an ocean beach, is to experience surrender to a force outside oneself—a powerful force that can hold danger as well as nurture and pleasure.

The birth process has its own rhythms, and some women have compared them to the sea. Surrender is the key to feeling safe in its embrace, and this is most possible when you have faith in the positive outcome of your efforts. Believing that a power greater than human power safeguards your welfare can assure success.

Birth is a momentous achievement, a triumphant assertion of the power of life itself. You can approach it as a battle to be won or as a cooperative endeavor; battles can be lost, but in cooperating everyone wins.

THOUGHT FOR TODAY: My need for understanding won't stand in the way of my surrender to forces outside my control.

Day 11

I had often occasion to notice the use that was made of fragments and small opportunities in Cranford; the rose-leaves that were gathered ere they fell to make into a potpourri for someone who had no garden; the little bunches of lavender flowers sent to strew the drawers of some town-dweller, or to burn in the chamber of some invalid.

—ELIZABETH GASKELL

In Gaskell's fictional world of a Victorian English village, nothing is wasted. Her characters are women whose lives are full of tiny crises and celebrations, and in which all possible elements are recycled, much like the fine texture of life itself.

In a healthy pregnancy, although you may not notice it, your body is using fragments and small opportunities, generating muscle tissue and blood vessels, busy with the work of metabolism, converting your substance into new compounds for use elsewhere—that is, in your baby's growing body.

If we wish to conserve our precious environment, we will learn from it. We can fertilize vegetables and flowers with our composted wastes. We can create our own pleasures and amusements from what we already have, rather than depending on further consumption. And like the citizens of Cranford, we can share what we have with those who do not have enough.

THOUGHT FOR TODAY: Shared wealth, like shared joy, further enriches the giver.

Day 12

Just as they perceive the light, unborn infants perceive the sounds of the world—despite the thickness of the mother's stomach wall.

They receive them the way fish do, through the waters in which they bathe. Sounds modulated, transformed.

And then birth!

—FREDERICK LEBOYER

Well, not birth for a while, yet. Nearly three more months of housing this creature who sees, hears, and moves about. During this month, your baby's brain develops the characteristic folds and convolutions that permit humans to store so much more information than any other species. It also acquires your antibodies, so that in the vital early weeks of life your baby will be immune to all the infections you're immune to.

Your baby has the ability to swallow now, too, and to breathe. It still resembles a fish in many ways, yet it is becoming a distinctly land-dwelling creature, despite the fact that its days are spent immersed in fluids.

During these months many pregnant women become increasingly introspective, though they may not spend much time consciously thinking of the growing independent life that accompanies them everywhere. It's almost as though you need more time for contemplation, before the bustling busyness of infancy commences.

THOUGHT FOR TODAY: I will treasure these months of growth, so that I can greet the next stage of my baby's life freely.

Day 13

. . . genius is as common as old shoes. Everybody has it, some more than others, perhaps, but that hardly matters, since no one can hope to use up more than a very small portion of his or her native gift.

—JOHN IRVING

The being who lives inside you now will be born with its own genius, its own endowment of intelligence, intuition, skills. Some kinds of ability do seem to be inborn; others seem to be wholly acquired; most seem to be part nature and part nurture.

All parents want their children to develop as fully as possible, to use their marvelous endowment in a way that makes them happy. It may seem mysterious to you now, but parents mostly need to get out of their children's way and let growth take its course. You'll want to make a wide spectrum of interests and opportunities available to your child, of course, but you can't control how these will be used.

No one can travel another's path, but one thing is certain: if you treat your child with respect, greeting it with unconditional love and making sure it knows you believe in its capacity to do whatever it wants to do, yours will be a happy, successful family.

THOUGHT FOR TODAY: I will do my best to prepare my child for joyful self-expression—and then let nature take its course.

Day 14

This is no rune nor symbol,
what I mean is—it is so simple

yet no trick of the pen or brush
could capture that impression . . .
— H.D.

Some scientists believe that all the imaging of the fetus that's now possible, beginning with the sonogram that you probably saw at ten weeks, is unnecessary. Sound waves have not been used medically for very long, and not much is known about their effects. Most practicing doctors and nurses believe they're harmless, but there simply is not enough evidence to prove one way or the other.

The main argument for not making images of the baby while it's in the womb, though, has to do with a sense of birth's holiness. Medical science has steadily decreased the secrecy and mystery of our physical processes, but perhaps it's not bad that some things are still hidden from the clinician.

Women know that our bodies sometimes communicate in ways that can't be expressed in language. Scientists tend to mistrust intuition and to look for hard evidence: x-ray photographs, scans, sonograms. When things go wrong, these can be useful; but in healthy pregnancy perhaps they shouldn't be allowed much importance.

THOUGHT FOR TODAY: My doctor or midwife works for me, and I can say what works for us.

Day 15

There are only two or three human stories, and they go on repeating themselves as fiercely as if they had never happened before.

—WILLA CATHER

Boredom is a concept totally foreign to our biology. If our cells grew weary with metabolizing, or if the constant repetition of secretion and synthesis were too much for our glands, human life would be a good deal different from what it is. Our hearts beat millions of times in an average life span; our neurons discharge millions, perhaps billions of electrical impulses. No, boredom belongs strictly to our consciousness, to human will.

For the most part, healthy adults manage to enjoy their lives even though much of our activity is repetitious. When sameness begins to grate on us, when we become bored or alienated, something's wrong. If you find that your routines seem drab, bleak, and uninviting, this could be a symptom of depression. You may want to seek counseling.

Late pregnancy is physically strenuous, and of course you're eager for the long-awaited birth. But when impatience becomes boredom, you don't need to suffer. You deserve to play your part with zest, finding radiance in your daily life.

THOUGHT FOR TODAY: Faith burnishes the details of my life. If they grow dull, I need to polish them up.

Day 16

Pregnancy can be a time of personal (not just fetal) growth and a precious, heightened phase in a woman's life. The key is personal balance; bringing your physical, emotional, mental and social sides into harmonious function.

—ELIZABETH DAVIS

When balance seems an impossible ideal, remember that you are not alone. Your spiritual guide, your connection to the source of all love and healing, is with you always, as close as your breath. Surrendering your preoccupations and praying for guidance will always improve the situation, even though serenity may still elude you: spiritual skills, like mental and physical ones, need to be developed and practiced.

Regular prayer and meditation will strengthen your spirit, as regular exercise strengthens your cardiovascular system. Think of spiritual practice as a cleansing procedure, one that sweeps away the inessentials that can clutter your mind. After cleaning, you can furnish your spirit as you choose, concentrating on the attitudes and responses that will be your most helpful companions: gratitude, love, detachment, surrender.

THOUGHT FOR TODAY: I can feed my spirit a balanced diet that will keep it fit and strong.

Day 17

Then to the Stars I flung my trust,
Scorning the menace of my coward dust;
Freed from my little will's control
To a good purpose marched my soul . . .
— Anna Wickham

Freeing yourself from the control of your "little will" is key to any program of spiritual growth. Our wills are part of our controlling desire that seeks to manage people and events. And our wills keep us chained to what we know, preventing us from exploring new possibilities.

When we can slip the leash of our little will and fling our trust upon a wider reality, we allow ourselves to discover spiritual wealth. Surrender of the will is such an important aspect of labor and delivery that if you have no experience of this letting go, pregnancy is a good time to acquire it.

You can use meditation to help you release your will. The same clean sweep effect results: once you let go of the desire for control, life becomes much more manageable. This miracle is due to faith in a power greater than ourselves, and the most direct route to that power is through surrender of the will.

THOUGHT FOR TODAY: All that stands between me and the gifts of faith is my will. I can choose to surrender it.

Day 18

> *We are learning by heart*
> *what has never been taught . . .*
> —AUDRE LORDE

For a woman whose pregnancy is difficult throughout its duration, cheerful platitudes are offensive. She needs sympathy and understanding, support for her courage, and recognition of her stamina. Few of us ever experience sustained physical hardship, and carrying a pregnancy to term when every movement requires conscious effort is a hardship.

Books, magazines, and advertisements trumpet the joys of pregnancy. It can seem cruelly unfair that a natural process should entail severe discomfort—nausea, sleep disturbance, fatigue, depression, or disorders of circulation. Yet what encourages a woman to continue is her strong desire for the new life to be born.

The last trimester of a difficult pregnancy tests a woman's spirit as well as her body. After months of discomfort your patience and serenity may lie in shreds. The discipline of meditation can help you to gain a wider perspective. Even a small improvement is an improvement.

THOUGHT FOR TODAY: My solution to discomfort is to concentrate on surviving each moment as it comes. By staying in the present, I can keep pregnancy joyful.

Day 19

"The best thing for disturbances of the spirit," replied Merlyn, beginning to puff and blow, "is to learn. That is the only thing that never fails."

—T. H. WHITE

An unexpected gift of this pregnancy can be learning—learning for yourself, as an adult, the theories and practices you need. Many women study the practice of deep breathing during their last months of pregnancy, using the method of French obstetrician Ferdinand Lamaze; they find deep breathing during labor lessens discomfort.

Dr. Lamaze's great idea was that one can't concentrate fully on two things simultaneously—as Merlyn says, one can't both learn and be disturbed. If a woman is wholeheartedly involved in the rhythm of her breathing, she cannot give herself to the cycle of pain, fear, and tension that increases the difficulty of labor.

It's an idea that works for millions of women. Acquiring a new discipline focuses our minds so that we don't give ourselves to small worries and preoccupations. Detaching from anxieties allows us to direct our energies more effectively. The Lamaze technique trains the body and quiets the spirit. Not every pregnant woman can find a Lamaze teacher or group, but everyone can find or order books to learn the technique.

THOUGHT FOR TODAY: Pregnancy can be a time of constant learning, constant refreshment of my mind and spirit so that they grow strong enough to withstand disturbances.

Day 20

It is astonishing how seldom things of this kind, which are apparently innerly determined, happen in the wrong place and at the wrong time. Six weeks earlier, I had spoken at Barnard's seventy-fifth anniversary celebration. When my former professor, Miss Howard, telephoned to ask whether I would do this, I said, "But I'm expecting a baby at about that time." Her response came crisply, "Well, you won't have it at the dinner, will you?"

—MARGARET MEAD

All pregnant women hear stories about emergency births, inconvenient labor, startling and dramatic circumstances—but these are really all rarities. Your hormones govern your physical responses to such a powerful degree that in the overwhelming majority of cases, labor doesn't begin at inappropriate moments.

Our biological processes are "innerly determined," but our bodies receive and integrate signals from our minds and spirits *and* from outside ourselves. Everyone agrees that emotions have biochemical effects, sometimes quite strong ones. Thoughts may reflect less intensely than feelings, but they too have a physical reality.

The closer you are to your due date, the fewer challenges you need. But if some ceremony requires your presence, don't refuse it because you're going to have a baby. Remember you are one person; your womb knows what the rest of you is doing.

THOUGHT FOR TODAY: Each day I receive more assurance that my being is integrated; body, mind, and spirit all becoming ready to give birth to this child.

Day 21

One of the mothers
the mother out of whose body
I easily appeared

Once I remembered her
— GRACE PALEY

In many families, women reckon their descent through the female line—mother, grandmother, great-grandmother. Sometimes infants are given names that recall this lineage. Birth stories are told and retold. As women's lives become more central in our thinking, pregnancy is more and more an opportunity to remember our mothers.

Many women mother children they have not borne; many of us have been mothered by several women. Your child will always be yours, but other mother figures will enter its life and memory.

"Women hold up half the sky" is a slogan from the Chinese women's movement that applies to our lives as well. Family patterns shift and blend; the realities of work, divorce, and day-care can interrupt a smooth continuity of mothers and children. But we can always remember to honor our mothers and all the other women who mother us and our children.

THOUGHT FOR TODAY: My baby and I are bonded by flesh and blood, but we will welcome all occasions for mothering.

Day 22

. . . I thought of how I would hold the baby, the new soft skin against my breast. My nipples would be the center of the baby's life, and my arms folding around the infant would fold around myself, holding the two of us together.

—ANNE ROIPHE

The emotional closeness of mother and newborn baby is unique in its beauty. From the intimacy and pleasure of this relationship, babies derive their earliest knowledge of love. We are blessed with this bond of need and nurture, although the mother-baby unity soon grows into a new relation, that of parent and child.

Many of us feel as adults that we had insufficient nurture when we were infants, and we promise ourselves that our babies will have enough. Perhaps we even fantasize that our babies can supply our deficit, providing the closeness our parents couldn't give.

We need to be clear: parents give their children emotional security, not the other way around. You have other resources for meeting your own needs, through intimacy with your partner, through therapy, and through learning to nurture yourself.

THOUGHT FOR TODAY: I can meet my baby's needs, because I'm able to get my own needs met.

Day 23

We need to dance the dance of life until we each are grown brave enough in its exultant beat to look into each other's eyes and chant our happiness, our joy, our courage in the face of death, our wish to live.

—KAREN MALPEDE

It takes strength of character to face each day, to occupy your life to the fullest extent possible, to truly be who you are. You may not feel much like dancing at this point in your pregnancy, but giving life is part of the dance, powerful encouragement we can give to others.

Courage can be acceptance of what comes, surrender to the inevitable. Our impulses to control our lives, to control other people, to schedule and predict and stay on top of things generally may be a refusal of courage. These impulses are frustrated in pregnancy, when it's so clear that in life we follow not our timetable but another, much vaster than we can comprehend, in which our cares and concerns are only one small part of the whole.

Simply by being what you are, you are dancing courageously right now, in the face of everything in the world that is sometimes inclined toward greed, oppression, cynicism, and despair. You are affirming joy.

THOUGHT FOR TODAY: I am brave because I do not seek to be other than I am.

Day 24

> *I had thought wisdom came with age*
> *that I had learned what I needed*
> *to move on with some grace*
> *if not with ease and dignity*
> *but mid-life years create me child*
> *again.*
>
> —JUDITH McDANIEL

Some women feel that they've definitely grown up when they're pregnant, and others discover a child within them that they never acknowledged before. Perhaps a part of you recalls being a baby in your own mother's womb; the experience of carrying a child in yours is so powerfully evocative that it's tempting to think perhaps the body's memories go back long before the conscious mind's.

Being in touch with your childish self needn't diminish the grace with which you conduct your life. Children play; children need nurture; within each of us, no matter how tall and serious we become, there lives a playful, needy child. Our intimate relationships are usually the outlet for our childish selves, because it's with our spouses and lovers that we dare to disclose our deepest desires. Pregnancy can be a time of special bonding for intimate partners, brought together by their shared needs for play and for nurture, stirred by their mutual consciousness of the new life they've created.

THOUGHT FOR TODAY: I need never be ashamed of my childish self; I will affirm her reality and nurture her within me.

Day 25

No gasp at a miracle that is truly miraculous because the magic lies in the fact that you knew it was there for you all along.

—TONI MORRISON

Nothing could be more truly miraculous than the presence of a baby within your body, a baby that has grown from two single cells, as all humans have done—you, your partner, your parents, the President; a baby that is already about a foot long and weighs about a pound and a half. Yet this miracle is such old stuff to you now that you hardly think about it. In a few short months, you've grown accustomed to this miracle.

What other miracles have occurred in your life? Perhaps you know friends or family members who have experienced miracles of faith, or who have found serenity in a miraculous release from chemical dependency. Perhaps someone close to you has experienced an extraordinary escape or recovery from some life-threatening condition. Such miracles take place daily. They are present in our lives, but we accept them, after our initial gratitude, as just another part of life. It's appropriate every now and then to acknowledge the miraculous and give thanks for it.

THOUGHT FOR TODAY: I will take heed of the miracles in my life and be grateful, for I know there will be more for me.

Day 26

Let nothing touched with evil,
Let nothing that can shrivel

Heart's tenderest friend, intrude
Upon your still, deep blood.
—STANLEY KUNITZ

Everyone has her own notion of what is evil; but for many people evil is associated with deprivation, with absence— instead of goodness and abundance of life, evil pinches, parches, and thwarts possibility. Being pregnant is the exact opposite of this. Life is lavish with you and your baby, and everything seems possible.

Many women say they never feel so *good*, morally speaking, as in pregnancy, and this feeling teaches them to recognize goodness wherever it's encountered. Generosity and abundance on the world stage deserve our admiration, and part of the goodness you can give your child is the knowledge that a better world is possible.

The child you have grown so carefully and well deserves a world of peace and plenty. Deep in its blood and spirit is the knowledge you can give it of what is good and what is evil; what must be accepted and what can be struggled for—or against.

THOUGHT FOR TODAY: My body knows that everything that nurtures life is good, and that my child will be born untouched by evil.

Day 27

I hope you will glisten with the glisten of ancient life, the same beauty that is in a leaf or a wild rabbit, wild sweet beauty of limb and eye.

—MERIDEL LeSUEUR

Human babies are wild animals when they're born, something their parents often forget. We think of wild creatures as being self-sufficient, fierce, and shy; babies are so helpless and cuddly, and they learn our ways so rapidly, that we can lose sight of the fact that at birth they're more like fawns or baby birds than like us.

Of course, they're wild animals with a difference: they have the equipment to be human beings, with language, technical proficiency, and moral judgments. Within little more than a year they will be comfortable in clothes, using spoons and cups, beginning to speak. But at first their responses will be wholly uncivilized.

Humans are nearly helpless at birth, and they need to stay for a long time in the warm nest, while their nervous systems acquire the vast amount of knowledge they must have to survive among us.

THOUGHT FOR TODAY: The sweet wild creature tames itself, when its parents give it warmth and touch.

Day 28

To quit was impossible once you had started.

All you could do was somehow to learn the ropes.

No one could teach you.

—Tom McGrath

All new parents have some moments of helpless panic when confronted with the actual fact of the baby they must care for. It's a job that's impossible to quit; somehow you have to learn the ropes, and even the best library and parents in the world can't teach you.

You know what you need to know, even though you may not believe it. Perfection is an ideal, not a human possibility; all parents make mistakes. New parents naturally want to avoid any mistakes they think their own parents made; but you'll undoubtedly make new ones, and your children will survive, just as you did.

Turn over your anxieties to a power greater than yourself. You have help in this vital project of caring for your baby, and you will succeed.

THOUGHT FOR TODAY: My baby is protected by the same power of creative love that safeguards me. We won't be allowed to stray too far.

Day 29

Once in a while she would cry for no reason, but the doctor said pregnant women do that.

—EILEEN MALONE

Your feelings are likely to be very close to the surface these days. Many women report that they laugh and cry more easily when they are pregnant and that they care more about things. Tears may spring to your eyes in response to minor frustrations, and small annoyances may provoke something close to hatred. You may be very surprised at your volatility.

"Pregnant women do that" for perfectly good reasons. Your hormonal system is functioning at an unprecedentedly high level, your glands secreting the substances that enable your body to carry out your creative, heroic task of bearing a child. Because human beings have such beautifully integrated circuitry, you can't turn down one set of responses while another is working so hard: all of you is working hard, your emotions no less than your body and spirit. You don't need to feel anything but proud of your strong feelings.

THOUGHT FOR TODAY: I deserve understanding from my support system, not impatience. There are perfectly good reasons for my responses.

Day 30

> *There is no predicting an American's future*
> *By the wealth or the people he was born amid*
> *He might grow up as the county moocher*
> *Or he might build a bridge on the lowest bid . . .*
> *He might go to Washington as Lincoln did.*
> —MATTHEW BILLER

As children most of us were encouraged to believe we could do anything we wanted to do. We weren't taught that our future is greatly affected by the social class we're born into. And we weren't taught how to help change the systems that thwart possibilities.

Can we do better for our children? We want them to keep a sense of limitless possibility, a belief that dreams can come true and that hard work and persistent vision can give anyone a good life. But we also want our children to understand the forces that keep some of us from realizing our potential, and to work to change them.

To work effectively for change, we must be able to bond with others and to balance our convictions with humility about what we don't know. Your faith in the world's possibilities coupled with your guidance will give your child a head start.

THOUGHT FOR TODAY: I will instill in my child the value of hard work and the self-confidence to make positive changes.

With you I ran
To see the roadside green
Leaves and small cool bindweed flowers
Living rejoicing to proclaim
We are, we are manifold, in multitude

We come, we are near and far,
Past and future innumerable, we are yours,
We are you . . .
—KATHLEEN RAINE

By reaching deep levels of relaxed concentration, you sometimes can touch a paradoxical sense of oneness with all creation. Alone and focused within yourself, you are suddenly exalted by the sense of multitudes. This outreaching consciousness, this universal love, is a gift of prayer and meditation especially precious in pregnancy.

Pregnant women are so focused on their new lives—the babies they carry, and the implications of those babies for their own future lives—that it's easy to lose a sense of connection with the rest of creation. A fresh look at a spring flower, an orange, a piece of music, or a stone can bring you back into harmony with the universe.

You and your baby occupy a special place in this closely woven collectivity. And the multitudes are important for you to love, too; their places create your place.

THOUGHT FOR TODAY: When my baby enters the world, the larger pattern will become more beautiful by the addition.

THIS MONTH'S VISIT TO THE DOCTOR

Date:

Weight: Blood Pressure:

Weight Gain:

This Month's Signs of Pregnancy:

Changes in Eating:

Changes in Sleeping:

Changes in Activities/Energy Level:

Reflections:

Questions for Next Month's Visit:

Day 1

This little light of mine,
I'm gonna let it shine,
Every day, every day, every day, every day,
Let my little light shine.
—African American Gospel song

Everyone who sees you knows that you're soon to be a mother. Are you finding that strangers tend to smile at you? This pregnancy is light-giving, because you're an image of hope: new life means new possibilities.

It's said, "The world is born fresh with every child." You will have the chance to see this fresh new world taking shape for your baby. This hope isn't a private one; it's for all of us. A pregnant woman is an image of all the possibilities that could belong to us.

A light shines forth from you, illuminating not only your path but the lives of everyone you meet. The new life is a beacon of hope, of continuity, and of salvation.

THOUGHT FOR TODAY: I cherish the hope that my child's life will be illuminated by peace and pleasure.

Day 2

"We can't hold on to each other like a piece of clothin'—puttin on and takin off when it suits us," Cora said impatiently, thinking of the unreliability of human relationships, especially those with kinfolk.

—CHERYL CLARKE

    Relationships with kinfolk can be unreliable. Twenty years from now, will you be sitting and wondering why this child doesn't call you?

    For now, your connection is only too reliable. Yet this new life will belong to a separate person, with faults and virtues that belong entirely to her or him. You may be your baby's entire world for the next months and even years, but it has its own path to follow, which will soon diverge from yours.

    The deep love you feel for your baby can help you to learn detachment, the healthy kind of detachment that will allow it to grow at its own pace, while you step gracefully out of the way. This love teaches that all creatures belong to themselves; that hanging on to someone or something is never good; that all life is change and all change is part of the great scheme of things, hidden from our individual eyes.

THOUGHT FOR TODAY: I may struggle against the flow of events, but wisdom and serenity counsel me to surrender. What I cannot understand, I'll strive to accept.

Day 3

More and more heavily, day by day
nature weighs down the mind.
A laziness like wisdom
overshadows the mouth with silence.
— BELLA AKHMADULINA

If "nature" were somehow separate from you, your body, your baby, and your mind, then you might agree that it's weighing you down. And it's true, in terms of strict avoirdupois, it is! But you are one integrated being. Consider this rather a change in you, in all of you, mind and body, heart and spirit.

The languor you may sometimes feel—a reluctance to move or speak, a contentment within yourself—has to do with your consciousness of the baby. As it takes up more of your body, it also occupies more of your spirit. When you don't know the answers to the questions that pose themselves, try to let the questions go.

It may be easier for you to meditate, these days. After months of practice, you may be able to reach a deep, relaxed meditative state even on a coffee break or while riding the bus. These precious intervals of calm, when you can simply be inside your skin with your baby, help you to free yourself of noise—uncertainties, nagging questions, doubts that can't be resolved.

THOUGHT FOR TODAY: I'm grateful for the gift of meditation; it's one I'll be able to use after my baby comes.

Day 4

Only if we become sensitive to the fine and subtle ways in which a child may suffer humiliation can we hope to develop the respect for him that a child needs from the very first day of his life onward, if he is to develop emotionally.

—ALICE MILLER

The new life deserves respect. Sometimes in pregnancy couples joke about the baby, teasing in order to lighten the effort; but after the baby comes, they're usually so softened and awed by the new creature that teasing is forgotten.

Under stress, the teasing behavior sometimes reappears. Now is the time to think at length about how you want to treat your child. Some teasing may be appropriate, when a child is old enough to share the joke, when it's clear that parents too can be teased. But mockery can be cruel to a small person, even a baby you might think is too young to understand.

Babies understand attitudes, and if your attitude is one of love and concern, that will be understood. You'll need to pay attention to your child, for everyone has different thresholds for humiliation—a remark that wounds one may be ignored by another. It's best not to risk the wound in the first place.

THOUGHT FOR TODAY: Even if my family tradition includes teasing, my baby deserves loving attention and respect.

Day 5

Can love remember
The question and the answer,
For love recover
What has been dark and rich and warm all over?
                                    —W.H. AUDEN

What we want most for our children is that they will have the capacity to give and receive love, and this we learn in our families. A child who is well loved, who is surrounded by adults who treat each other lovingly, has a sense of mutuality and will be capable of intimacy.

In all our intimate relationships we seek the "dark and rich and warm all over" knowledge of our earliest nurture—of life before birth, when everything we needed was given to us. Successful partners nurture each other, and a child who is raised in the confidence of unconditional love will be a successful partner.

THOUGHT FOR TODAY: Whether I'm rich or poor, I can love lavishly, unstintingly, and my baby can receive this gift of my spirit.

Day 6

Balzac . . . described creation in terms of motherhood. Yes, in an intelligent passionate motherhood there are similarities, and in more than the toil and patience. The calling upon total capacities; the reliving and new using of the past; the comprehensions; the fascination, absorption, intensity.
—TILLIE OLSEN

In pregnancy you are involved in a great work of the cosmic imagination, and it has a lot in common with the bringing forth of a great work of art. Everything in your life is brought to bear on this pregnancy. Even character traits or events from your past that you may dislike or find unproductive can be transformed into useful aspects of your character.

Every human attribute exists on a continuum, and you can choose how your attributes will affect your life. If you've been impatient or headstrong, you can find courage. If you have been timid or unresponsive, these defects can be transformed to yield caution and patience.

You are your first great creative work; your baby is your second. Everything you learn about yourself will yield dividends.

THOUGHT FOR TODAY: Each day gives me an opportunity for creative expression, and I will use it as best I can.

Day 7

> *For part of its rest, the*
> *infant must be put down.*
> —MARTY ROTH

For most of us, the people in our lives are far more precious than our possessions—ideas, beliefs, or property. Our joy and also our anguish come from our relationships, and we find that generally we receive love and concern in the same proportion as we give them to others.

Parenthood is a new kind of relationship. Extraordinary demands will be made on you, for patience, tolerance, fortitude, and sometimes sheer physical endurance; but the rewards are beyond anything in your experience. One of the rewards is the self-knowledge that parenting yields.

The spiritual force that powers our lives teaches us the importance of love. This power also lets us know that respect is an integral part of love; we're not fully loving if we transgress another's intimate boundaries. An essential part of parents' love is letting children grow into their own lives.

THOUGHT FOR TODAY: Loving is a vital part of my own program for spiritual growth, and letting go is part of loving.

Day 8

If men did equally share in parenting, it would mean trading places with women part of the time. Many men have found it easier to share power with women on the job than they have in the home.

—MARY ELLEN SCHOONMAKER

The mother-infant bond is so tremendously strong that fathers sometimes feel left out, beginning in late pregnancy. You and the baby form an indissoluble pair. Even in a relationship that has always been an equal one, the father may feel that neither of you really needs him. These feelings may be unconscious, but they're powerful nonetheless.

Through touch and smell fathers can form as vital a bond with the baby as mothers. If fathers care for their babies physically from the very beginning—changing diapers, giving baths, carrying the baby in a sling—they'll feel more power as parents. What can interfere with this father-baby bond is the mother's resentment at her powerlessness in other aspects of family life.

Too often, power struggles between parents are played out in the lives of children. Parents may not realize what they're doing, but if the mother discourages the father from full partnership, everyone loses. The key is confidence in your own power, and trust in your partner to share equally.

THOUGHT FOR TODAY: I can only share what I have. If I feel powerless, I must claim power over my life.

Day 9

Emotion is as old as life, but the intellect is so young that it
must be cherished. And it is precious enough to cherish.
—AGNES SMEDLEY

The strong feelings that sweep through you don't always
direct your actions; you have a choice about how you behave
in response to any given situation. Feelings may impel you in
directions that your intellect rejects; you may feel like a small
child yourself, at times, when life calls on you for adult
responses.

Feelings can't be ignored, though they needn't always be
acted upon. But it's important to acknowledge them. When
you feel vulnerable and needy, you can ask for nurture, from
your partner or from your higher power. Your feelings are
always right for you, because you have them, but they need
not always guide your actions.

If you can acknowledge your feelings, you can choose
how they influence your behavior. This balance of intellect
and feeling is one key to serenity.

THOUGHT FOR TODAY: I will be a better parent if I can
admit that sometimes I feel as needy as a child. When I am
connected to a source of spiritual nourishment, all my needs
can be met.

> *Mother I am*
> *Identical*
> *With infinite Maternity*
> > *Indivisible*
> > *Acutely*
> > *I am absorbed*
> > *Into*
> *The was-is-ever-shall-be*
> *Of cosmic reproductivity*
> > > —MINA LOY

Are you in danger of forgetting who else you are, besides this about-to-be mother? There is more in your life than bearing and mothering, though you've been so concentrated on this coming event for so long that even your unconscious, dreaming mind seems possessed by it.

Inner reflection lets you know that you're bringing your whole self to this birth. Your child will be born from your mind and heart as well as from your body; also, you'll be giving birth to a new identity for yourself: mother.

You're not in control of these birthings, though you're at their center. Meditation helps you surrender control willingly, and surrendering control keeps you in balance.

THOUGHT FOR TODAY: My baby and I are participating fully in this work of creation, and we are partnered by sympathetic forces.

Day 11

I like thinking that she's going to become a new member of our community—that she's being born into an existing group of friends.

—PAT DOWELL

The best reason to have a baby shower is for friends to gather to demonstrate their welcome for a coming child, to offer tokens of their faith that a new valuable member will be added to their community. Friends signal their willingness to expand their affections. They bring gifts to comfort and sustain mother and baby, and eat and drink in your honor.

In this way you can look forward to your baby's growing up among your friends and their children, sharing your rituals, values, and observances. The baby will enrich your culture by helping you discover how to introduce a new member to it.

Your relationships will change, inevitably, as you enter this new phase of life, and your understanding will deepen. Your baby is making a mother out of you, and your view of the world is changing subtly as it shows you new possibilities.

THOUGHT FOR TODAY: Rituals of welcome for my baby also welcome me in my new role.

Day 12

Consider the facts, we said. First there are nine months before the baby is born. Then the baby is born. Then there are three or four months spent in feeding the baby. After the baby is fed there are certainly five years spent in playing with the baby. You cannot, it seems, let children run about the streets.

—VIRGINIA WOOLF

Although Virginia Woolf had no children, she was acutely conscious that many women are caught in a painful dilemma: whether to pursue active professional lives or have children. Upper-class English women in her time turned the care of their children over to nursemaids, or nannies (and still do); of course, skilled day-care might have freed the lives of middle-class and working-class mothers, as well.

Most industrial democracies make day-care a matter of important social policy, since most mothers must work in the labor market as well as in the home. In many countries there are workplace nurseries, where mothers can nurse their babies or eat and play with their older children. In the United States, many women delay childbearing until they can afford a furlough from professional activity, but others are caught in the same bind.

Most mothers are on their own to find private care of some kind. A few employers provide good day-care in the workplace for mothers and fathers alike, promoting equality both at work and in child care.

THOUGHT FOR TODAY: Whatever child-care arrangements I'm able to make should benefit my whole family.

Day 13

Integrity is wholeness, the greatest
beauty is
Organic wholeness, the wholeness of life and things, the
divine
beauty of the universe.
—ROBINSON JEFFERS

For the baby, birth represents a break in continuity, the abrupt introduction to a new stage of life, but for you birth is the expected culmination of this long process. Just as you can see buds swelling in late winter with the life that will burst forth in spring, so your life has been preparing for the introduction of a new life inside it, soon to be beside it.

Nothing could be more natural than having a baby, yet for most of us birth signals a huge change. Most women feel anxious about their ability to care for their babies, because most of us have had little preparation. During this month, try to regain a sense of the wholeness of your experience. Your body has prepared for this baby since before you yourself were born, and you have everything you need to care for it.

THOUGHT FOR TODAY: My anxieties are unnecessary. I'll know what to do with my baby, and what I don't know, I can turn over to the wisdom of my spiritual guide.

Day 14

Children can't be a center of a life and a reason for being.
They can be a thousand things that are delightful, interesting,
satisfying, but they can't be a wellspring to live from.
—Doris Lessing

We've all seen people whose lives are diminished by inappropriate attachments to their parents or their children—families in which parents and children are so enmeshed in their attempts to "live from" each other that neither can use their personal powers. This cannot happen to people who have a sense of balance within themselves. Letting go of both your wishes and your fears will safeguard you against loading your family members with expectations they cannot fulfill.

Of course, your baby may well be the center of your life for some weeks or months. But before long, the claims of your own life, personality, and relationships will assert themselves. You'll be a better mother and a happier woman when your energies are deployed evenly in your life.

THOUGHT FOR TODAY: I can strike a balance in my life between family, work, friendships, and personal growth, and my baby will ultimately benefit.

Day 15

> *Miracles occur,*
> *If you care to call those spasmodic*
> *Tricks of radiance miracles. The wait's begun again,*
> *The long wait for the angel,*
> *For that rare, random descent.*
>
> —SYLVIA PLATH

What we call miracles can sometimes be very simple—the miracle of conception, the miracle of your baby's growth inside you. These wondrous things all happen so easily, with no particular fanfare or beating of wings, that we can easily overlook their splendor. It's only afterward that we feel the radiance.

Another miracle is within your reach these days—the miracle of letting go of your baby. She or he is a separate person, different from you, and life asks you to relinquish any sense that you own him or her.

You can imagine this letting-go, though you may not have achieved it yet. All you need to do is make yourself entirely ready for the miracle; when it's ready to happen, it will.

THOUGHT FOR TODAY: I can surrender myself to the breathing rhythms of life, taking in and letting out, holding on and letting go.

Day 16

It is possible that in some future generation, childrearing will be seen as the crucial activity of a culture, and the raising of future generations will be the most prized and rewarded profession.

—JUDY CHICAGO

Imagine a world in which power and respect are given to nurses, mothers, primary-school teachers, and day-care workers. They make decisions about how to spend the national wealth and order social priorities. It's safe to say that rather than planning to conquer other countries or to colonize space, our energies as a people would be directed toward developing our children's potential.

Policy debates would center on the best ways to prepare children for adult life. The health of women and babies would be crucial, much more important than the health of corporations; in fact, corporations might cease to exist, if the wise and powerful found they weren't contributing to the goals of society.

Just imagine for a moment what it might be like to live in a culture whose leaders actively valued life over property. It's light years away from where we are now, but who is to say it's not possible to get from here to there?

THOUGHT FOR TODAY: I can choose the vision that guides me, and I can pray for the wisdom to help it come about.

Day 17

Me, in bed, a rectangle of light through the open door. Her scent; her laugh. A streetlight shines through my curtains, or is it a moon? Snow muffles the traffic. Quiet outside; secrets within.

—Alice Silverman

Do you have memories from early childhood of your mother, all dressed up and smelling wonderful? Was she the moon and stars to you? I used to feel a current of delicious sadness running underneath my love and admiration for my mother, sadness at the parts of her life that had nothing to do with me. My mother could change from her ordinary weekday self who went to work and came home, made toast for breakfast and lamb chops for dinner, kissed me and scolded me, read to me and tucked me in; she could go dancing in black chiffon and opals.

You are the whole world to your baby, and you will be for quite a while. Your child first learns about possibility from you. This is a serious responsibility, but it's also a source of joy; very little in life can compare with the look of utter love and trust in your baby's eyes.

Your touch is your baby's whole experience. Very soon, other experiences will crowd in, but you'll remain your baby's principal connection to the world. What strong connections you possess, your baby will, too.

THOUGHT FOR TODAY: My life includes dancing along with drudgery, beauty along with the pain. My baby will understand the dangers and learn from them, too.

Day 18

> *Each mortal thing does one thing and the same:*
> *Deals out that being indoors each one dwells;*
> *Selves—gives itself;* myself *it speaks and spells,*
> *Crying* What I do is me: for that I came.
> —GERARD MANLEY HOPKINS

Newborn flowers don't cry, or newborn crabs, or earth-worms. They manage to speak and spell themselves in ways that are much less wracking to our nerves than an infant's fussing or yelling. But the being that dwells inside them asks much less from their species. No geranium needs to learn English or to eat with a fork; shellfish never need to learn to count or tie their shoes.

What they do is be themselves, simply and wholly, and what your baby will do is what it came for: to grow, with your help, into the best human being possible. Crying and fussing are part of growth, an expression of each baby's individual relation to its family and its world.

Some infants seem much more demanding than others; one baby never naps for more than twenty minutes at a time and howls for a couple of hours every night, while another sleeps peacefully and lives quietly when awake. These differences don't seem to have any correlation to how these children will grow. The noisy one could easily become a cloistered mystic and the quiet one a rock musician.

THOUGHT FOR TODAY: Trust in the wisdom of forces I can't see will help me accept my baby's constantly changing identities.

Day 19

When newly born, a baby cries at the slightest frustration because up until now all its needs have been completely met. . . . It has never been cold, hungry or lonely. There is no way it can know that you are nearby in the next room, or that you will nurse it "as soon as you get off the phone."
—ELIZABETH DAVIS

Drawing on your deep physical sympathy with your baby's needs, you understand that it has almost everything to learn. If you find yourself expecting a new baby to tell time or read your mind, you have moved away from the place of mutual understanding. In our bodies, we carry the deep memory of infancy, and your months of pregnancy can refresh this memory for you.

Most of this sympathy is outside your control, of course, and will continue to be—for example, your milk may let down at the baby's cry; you may wake at subtle changes in its breathing. All this openness and sympathy can get in the way of household life. New mothers find their attention severely strained in the early weeks, between the baby's needs and their own.

Be gentle and generous with yourself, your partner, and your baby. If you allow yourself to be the loving, well-meaning, imperfect parent that you are, you may discover reserves of patience with your baby's needs. All too soon, your child will learn the difficult facts of life outside the womb. Hold onto your serenity, and all will be well.

THOUGHT FOR TODAY: My baby learns about the world from me. Is it a place where needs are met, or is it a place of frustration, anger, and despair? The difference lies greatly within my power.

Day 20

> *I reach the summit*
> *And gradually subside into anticipation of*
> *Repose*
> *Which never comes.*
> *For another mountain is growing up*
> *Which   goaded by the unavoidable*
> *I must traverse*
> *Traversing myself*
>
> —MINA LOY

Your doctor or midwife may have told you you'd be sleeping more lightly, waking more often, in these last months. Even if you're tired during the day, most pregnant women find they sleep less, dreaming lightly, skimming the surface of sleep. It's almost as though your body is practicing endurance, gearing up for the major work of bringing forth your baby.

Be glad you've taken such good care of yourself, eating wisely, doing your breathing exercises, keeping as fit as you can. In many ways, labor resembles an athletic event. You might think you could never do a triathlon, but your body is preparing for an ordeal that will equal one in intensity and may take a good deal longer.

Athletes have talked and written of the self-knowledge they gain from pitting themselves against great odds. You can expect the same from your coming adventure. Your body literally was made for this; you won't be given more than you can handle.

THOUGHT FOR TODAY: From traversing the peaks, I earn the valleys. By climbing the slope, I achieve the next peak.

Day 21

. . . there are as many fine children born out of the more despicable emotions—boredom, spite, anger, pique, frustration, envy, gall, spleen, and sheer absent-mindedness—as ever were born out of love or desire.

—ANTHONY THORNE

Many parents harbor lingering guilt over their imagined failures, even before their first child is born. The circumstances of conception may have been less than ideal; perhaps in early pregnancy you took risks; illness or trouble during pregnancy may have spoiled the serenity you sought. Rest assured, very little of this will make any difference to your baby.

One would like to have a blissful, perfect moment of conception and nine months of positive thinking to prepare one's offspring. Unfortunately, life's not like that. A couple who are trying to plan a pregnancy may get so stressed that lovemaking becomes a chore. In the course of even the most ardently desired pregnancy there are down times, sicknesses, regrets. None of this interferes with the terrific strength of the life force that will send your baby out of your body into the waking world.

THOUGHT FOR TODAY: When I think about it, any regrets or second thoughts I have will vanish in the anticipation of my baby's birth.

Day 22

> *Spirit enters flesh*
> *And for all it's worth*
> *Charges into earth*
> *In birth after birth*
> *Ever fresh and fresh.*
> —Robert Frost

The word *spirit* describes what makes us human, the spark that relates us to other human beings and to the world. What's amazing is that although *spirit* could also be said to be that part of us that doesn't change—unlike flesh, which gets pregnant, delivers, grows, matures, and dies—it is forever new.

Forever new and forever loving and trusting, whatever happens to the rest of us. Our minds and hearts may become jaded or hardened, but our innermost spirit remains bright. And we can always pray through it; the spirit survives any adventures of the body and mind.

Renewal thus is always within your reach, for it dwells in you. The solution to every problem, the balm for every wound, your connection to the timeless source of love and healing always responds to prayer.

THOUGHT FOR TODAY: I can't control what happens to me, but I'm sovereign of myself. Everything I want for myself and my baby is within my reach.

Day 23

We teach our children one thing only, as we were taught: to wake up.

—ANNIE DILLARD

New parents wait eagerly for their babies to recognize them, to wake up. Babies learn the world through their parents. Your familiar face, voice, smell, and touch will introduce your baby gently to the techniques of living. The gifts you possess, you will bestow on your child.

In dealing with your baby, patience and humility may bring you close to memories from your own infancy, from the time before you woke up; many new mothers are surprised at the complexity of their responses to their babies' cries. "I felt that it was me crying," one friend said. "So I tried to comfort myself while I was nurturing my child."

We're all former babies, and deep inside each of us is a place where we understand the difficulties of adjusting to independent life. This sympathetic place is like a clearing in the forest; our habits have grown up around it, but we can penetrate to its openness, and it will keep us gentle.

THOUGHT FOR TODAY: While rearing a future grown-up, I'll remember that I'm a former infant.

Day 24

I could feel my blood like a river inside me, and my breast deep and thigh and womb ready for a new child, and strong labor for it and I liked it.

—Meridel LeSueur

Women are familiar with blood, from our menstrual periods. The fact that birth is a bloody event doesn't shock most women or upset them. Blood is the fluid of life; the spirit of destruction is very close to the creative spirit, for they are two ends of the same vital cord.

Yet some men feel squeamish, when they learn that their offspring will first appear bearing traces of their partners' blood. Old, involuntary responses can kick in. Underneath their warm feelings of sympathy and support for you, they may fear losing control. Some doctors are reluctant to let fathers attend births, even though in many hospitals it's standard practice.

If your partner feels at all ambivalent about being present in the delivery room, the two of you should discuss procedures with your doctor or nurse. Some fathers are eager to help, for example, to cut the umbilical cord; others want to photograph the event, or simply to experience it. Some really don't want to be present. Keeping communication open between you, you'll arrive at the level of participation that's right for you.

THOUGHT FOR TODAY: My baby's father has his own relationship to the coming birth. I'll do my best to see that he is happily involved in our baby's birth.

Day 25

*It's amusing to see how, even on my microscopic field, minute
events are perpetually taking place illustrative of the broadest
facts of human nature.*

—ALICE JAMES

Each one of us sees only a "microscopic field," yet our
minute events make up the larger picture. The birth of your
baby will be unique, and at the same time typical: it will take
its place within the sequence of births, growths, and transfor-
mations.

Every woman has unique experiences in labor and birth,
yet we have these in common with all other women who are
mothers. Each smallest detail of your experience has been
shared by some other woman, at some time, and other women
can learn from you. Your baby's new life is at the same time
infinitely precious and as common as grass.

You and your baby will set your individual stamp on
labor, birth, and infancy. In your daily life the small events
will echo in the lives of others, on a different scale. Nothing is
new under the sun, except you in this moment of your life.

THOUGHT FOR TODAY: I take comfort in our kinship with
all mothers and babies, and pride in our individuality.

Day 26

The baby should be addressed in its own language. The language that precedes words.

Are we, then, to speak in gestures, as we would to a foreigner? Of course not.

We must go back still further and rediscover the universal language, which is simply the language of love.

—FREDERICK LeBOYER

Someone once told me the best way to learn another language is to have a lover who doesn't speak your own; then you are motivated to find ways to communicate. Although your baby can't be said to know a different language, you both are motivated to find clear communication within your intimacy.

In the early days and weeks, you'll find *touch* is the most basic means of communication. A soothing massage conveys love and healing more powerfully than any words. Cold fingers, an unsure grip, hurried or awkward movements communicate discomfort and anxiety. Some insecurity is inevitable; you may never have cared for a new infant, and of course you're anxious not to drop or harm it. Trust the baby as you want it to trust you, and you'll soon master the art of communication.

THOUGHT FOR TODAY: If I pray for guidance, any anxieties will be eased. I'll recover the lost language of loving touch with my baby.

Day 27

. . . I imagine the inside of my body
glowing, phosphorescent, with strange flower faces . . .
                                    —DIANE WAKOSKI

The placenta and membranes now make up only about one-third of the contents of your uterus—much less than in earlier months. They've been surpassed by your baby, who is rapidly gaining weight.

If your baby were to be born now, it would have excellent chances for completely normal delivery and development. The most important work of its growth is done. There may be days when you wish heartily for an early birth; on other days you may dread the prospect of giving birth to this large creature still inside you.

Labor is triggered by a sequence of hormone secretions, and no one knows exactly what signal releases them. The body responds to its own mysterious signals. The intravenous drip that is sometimes given to hasten labor contains a synthetic form of the hormone oxytocin that your body makes naturally. The medication that's given to slow an early labor also contains it. When the time comes, you may or may not need a drip. Despite all this language of "early" and "late," by and large, your body is taking good care of you and your baby.

THOUGHT FOR TODAY: I don't have to understand the chemistry of pregnancy, just accept and collaborate with it.

Day 28

"Henry Rackmeyer, you tell us what is important."
"A shaft of sunlight at the end of a dark afternoon, a note in music, and the way the back of a baby's neck smells . . ."
"Correct," said Stuart. "Those are the important things."
—E. B. WHITE

It is so easy for our priorities to become confused. We tend to think that "the important things" are material— municipal bonds, real estate, the national debt. Our lives are affected far more intimately by the events of our senses. Not that the large things aren't important, but we can't change them. We may choose to direct our energies to long-term change, as in politics or banking, but the here and now is where we live.

Great changes in our lives may be wrought by irreversible events like birth and death, but day to day our lives are sustained by small repeated changes in light, sound, smell, taste, touch, and what we choose to do with them. We have intellectual and spiritual power to transform those small, important things in our lives. We can choose to dwell in comfort and pleasure, nourished by—for example—the clean smell of a baby's neck, or we can separate ourselves from them.

THOUGHT FOR TODAY: My baby will be born into my here and now. I'll do my best to make a life worthy of it.

Day 29

Can you guess how many rice plants we have?

Do you know how many tributaries the river has?

Who can sweep all the leaves in the forest?
                                                    —Tran Thi Nga

    Folk songs and poems about babies often take the form of riddles, as though the only way we have of grasping the mystery of birth is through this kind of word magic. We know we are numerous as the sands of the sea or the leaves in the forest, yet we're uniquely precious to one another.

    The essence of a mystery is that it cannot be understood. You will learn to understand your little kicking mystery, to accept that it is both you and not-you, both animal and human, tough and fragile, the same and different.

    The downy hair that covered your baby's body in earlier months is disappearing now, although you may see some evidence of it at birth. The gills through which it breathed when it was very tiny have been transformed through its development into glandular structures in the neck. Its spine no longer ends in a tail. It's a human baby, but it has traveled far through mysterious realms of growth to reach you in its present state.

THOUGHT FOR TODAY: I can follow my baby's travels in imagination, and I'll be grateful for its safe arrival.

Day 30

When I talk with friends who have struggled with addictions to alcohol or cigarettes or with eating disorders, I always feel that the answer is to get to be an insider in your body, respond to the signals it gives about what will make it feel right.
—RUTH HUBBARD

Those of us who have struggled with addictions and are recovering from them know that this is good advice, but we also know there is something that must come first, a beginning before the beginning. In order to trust the signals of our bodies, we must believe we have a right to health. A great deal of misery stems from feelings of unworthiness, feelings that we don't deserve the best that life can give.

Recovery from a spiritual sickness is not a single event but a continuing process—continuing, for many of us, throughout our lives. Whether our addiction was to a substance or a mode of thinking—addiction to despair, to crisis, or to another person—our recovery takes place as we learn to behave positively, creatively, life-affirmingly.

We must learn to hear our bodies' signals before we can teach ourselves to trust them, and in this endeavor we have a constant source of guidance. A spiritual connection to a source of power greater than ourselves can protect us so we can find healing.

THOUGHT FOR TODAY: My baby and I deserve the best of everything, and the tools for obtaining the best are within our grasp.

Day 31

A door stands open in the heart
And all good things are true.
—WILLIAM ROSE BENÉT

If you have been practicing meditation or prayer, or both, throughout the months of your pregnancy, you've learned to open that door in your heart. Life is a complex web, and we automatically screen out most of its influences, but prayer asks us to open ourselves again to the flood of goodness and truth.

When we can do this, truly all good things are possible. We're centered, able to tap the source of spiritual power that blesses our endeavors. If you don't achieve this surrender of the will in a month, or six months, or even six years, don't give up. Spiritual discipline is the work of a lifetime, even more so than growing and nurturing your child.

What you learn from this pregnancy and birth will enrich your spirit forever, as your spiritual growth up to now has enriched your pregnancy. You bring everything you are to each moment of your life, and you need never stop growing.

THOUGHT FOR TODAY: I am opening my spirit, as my body will open to give birth to my child.

THIS MONTH'S VISIT TO THE DOCTOR

Date:

Weight: Blood Pressure:

Weight Gain:

This Month's Signs of Pregnancy:

Changes in Eating:

Changes in Sleeping:

Changes in Activities/Energy Level:

Reflections:

Questions For Next Visit:

Day 1

I had had help in the child's conception, but no one could deny that I had had an immaculate pregnancy.

—MAYA ANGELOU

Here begins your last month in the same body as your baby. Even though birth may come a few days after the date you've fixed on, this is the final stretch. You've used this opportunity to strengthen your spiritual connection, while your circumference widened and your baby perfected its growth.

Your pregnancy has been immaculate, because you and your baby have carried through with it together, bravely and innocently. Nothing you've done in these months has harmed you, or anyone else; it's a totally constructive process, totally creative. This may well be the most positive endeavor you've ever been part of, and through it many women come to love themselves in a new way.

You have discovered your power to create and nurture new life. Through all your baby's changes, all its fishy swimming and bumping around inside, it has shown you that you're a much bigger and better person—especially bigger— then you ever dreamed you could be.

THOUGHT FOR TODAY: Through this immaculate pregnancy I've discovered a beautiful new power, which I'll continue to nurture long after my baby is born.

Day 2

happen.

to

up

stacking

is

something

when nothing is happening

—MAY SWENSON

This poet was writing about the waves of the sea, not the birth process, yet her words are appropriate. Your baby's arrival is stacking up to happen, as surely as if it were a plane waiting to land. It will come from inside you, yet you won't really know it until after you're separated.

Remember always that there's never *nothing* going on. Events as great as your baby's birth are stacking up to happen all the time, and the people involved in them are caught up as you are and can't really explain the meaning of these happenings. Whatever happens will happen; our task is to trust in the power of love to bring about a good outcome.

THOUGHT FOR TODAY: Love made us partners in the first place, and love will safeguard our future relationship.

Day 3

Women learn to like themselves in the mothering roles, which allow them experiences of love and power not easily found in other situations.

—LINDA GORDON

Are all systems of authority based on the parent-child relationship? Sometimes it seems they are—education, religion, law enforcement, government, all these authorities recall our earliest relations to power: the parents into whose hands and households we were delivered.

You'll be aware, after your baby is born, of the enormous power you have been given, and it may both delight and scare you. To like yourself in the mothering role, you'll need to learn to use your power respectfully. Now and for a little while longer you are the whole world for your baby. It's within your power to choose the kind of world your baby encounters, and the higher the quality of your experience, the better you'll like yourself.

Your greatest power will be to empower your baby. As you grow together, you can help your child to become the loving presence it was meant to be.

THOUGHT FOR TODAY: My baby's gift to me is the knowledge of my power, and I can return it in kind. The strongest power is the power of love.

Day 4

In Japan she was made as happy to see carrots and lettuce growing in the fields as she was to see sunlight, years earlier, pouring into the streets of New York City. Everywhere she's been she's seen people eating and sleeping and working and making things with their hands and urging things to grow.
—CAROL SHIELDS

Anywhere in the world, you would be recognized for what you are, no matter how strange your language and culture to the people around you. Birth is a major event in everyone's life, and all societies have rules for birthing and caring for new mothers. In one sense, this care is as ordinary as sunlight, or garden vegetables; yet they are miraculous, too.

The simplicity of life's important things can make you happy, if you let yourself feel it deeply. You are protected by a power greater than yourself, the same power that urges things to grow in countries all over the globe. All human beings are united in our capacity to nurture new life, and our kinship is a cause for rejoicing.

THOUGHT FOR TODAY: If things seem too complex and threaten to overwhelm me, I can remember how simple goodness is, and I'll be comforted.

Day 5

> *The ship of life will push out of you*
> *and rejoice*
>   *in the whiteness,*
>
>   *in the first floating and rising of water.*
>   —KATHLEEN FRASER

Most of your body is composed of water, as is most of your baby's. It is still a little aquatic creature floating inside you, in a liquid environment. Your different fluids are separated by just a membrane. Because we all begin our lives in a sac of fluid inside our mothers, water is usually thought of as female.

In dreams, water can stand for women, or birth, or one's mother—and a newborn is often compared to a ship. There have been times, on this long voyage, when your baby may have felt more like heavy cargo in your hold than a ship of its own.

Birth is your baby's launching. It will sail under its own power, the flag of its own identity, and with you it will learn to navigate the rough seas as well as the calm. Remember, you are both guided by a source of illumination stronger than any lighthouse, which will see you both into safe harbor.

THOUGHT FOR TODAY: My baby feels the movement of my walking and breathing, just as I feel the rippling of waves when I'm on water.

Day 6

Life is like an add-a-pearl necklace. You don't stop being thirty when you turn thirty-one.

—Henry Ward

I can remember not wanting anything to change, in the ninth month of my first pregnancy. I felt—in addition to my unwieldy body and shortness of breath—serene and whole, to the point where I almost dreaded the birth. I knew so well how to be pregnant. The process had gone on long enough for me to get very good at it, and I didn't know nearly as well how to be the mother of my baby.

But I found out. Blessedly, I found that I could bring some of the serenity of late pregnancy with me into motherhood. All I lost was weight; my spiritual growth was steady. It's natural to dread this change, but remember, you know more than you think about mothering your child. All the disciplines you have practiced during pregnancy have strengthened your spirit. You're a more loving, caring person now than you were nine months ago, and you'll never lose those strengths if you don't choose to.

THOUGHT FOR TODAY: I can let go of what I don't choose to bring with me on my journey, and I can take along everything of value.

Day 7

> *. . . the power of relinquishing*
> *what one would keep; that is freedom . . .*
> —MARIANNE MOORE

All our lives most of us have been told—to the point of boredom—that true freedom requires discipline. Freedom is not easy, and it is never achieved by taking the path of least resistance. Those of us who are recovering from various addictions can testify to the truth of this axiom: the power to say no liberates us from a condition close to bondage.

In pregnancy, "relinquishing" belongs to a different sort of power. You don't so much *choose* to let go of your baby as you allow yourself to be carried along by your labor, to participate fully in a process greater than yourself. Yet it feels like freedom, this acquiescence to the tremendous power of birth.

Your body's capacity to bear and to bring forth a new life is miraculous. Your baby's birth will be its first step along an independent path, where you will help guide its steps. And birth will give you back the freedom of single tenancy in your own body; rejoice in its power.

THOUGHT FOR TODAY: I'll be able to enjoy my freedom, for I've disciplined my spirit and my body in preparation for this birth.

Day 8

I remember after the birth of one of my children a moment of uncontrollable laughter at the thought of how hopelessly final it all was. This baby who had been provided for so involuntarily inside me was now outside, forcing me into responsibility. Nothing was automatic any more.

—NANCY CALDWELL SOREL

For new parents the finality of their child's birth is alarming, although most pregnant women welcome the end of involuntary nurture. Once your baby is born you can enter into its life in a way you couldn't before. Your actions will have consequences for your baby, though no one can say exactly what those consequences will be.

There is no blueprint or program for raising children. No one really understands how to do it, but most new parents manage with some success. You have the advantage of your own spiritual program to guide you through these uncharted territories, and though birth is certainly final, you are not alone in bearing responsibility. A higher power stands ready, as close as the deepest wish of your heart, to offer help with every aspect of your new life.

THOUGHT FOR TODAY: I plan to enjoy the challenge of nursing and rearing my baby as much as I've enjoyed growing it.

Day 9

I am honored to be in the presence of
the Expecting Mother. . . .
Your eyes are those of a Young Spirit looking
outward.
I thank the Creator for this Gift of Birth that we
as a People may continue tomorrow.
                                    —LEONARD MARTIN

The writer is a native American Indian, and his greeting to a new life puts it in the context of the continuity and survival of a people. Your baby will take its place among your people. However you celebrate the birth of a new member, it's an important occasion, when culture is extended forward in time.

All cultures have some prayers or ceremonies for welcoming new babies. Whether or not you choose a traditional naming or baptism, you can create a ritual that satisfies you and affirms your baby's place in the life of your family.

The important part is that it should have meaning for you. Planting a tree; composing a song; laying down a cask of wine; preparing and eating special foods; these all are meaningful rituals of welcome in various cultures. Make your affirmation as simple or elaborate as you like, but find some way to welcome the new life into your family.

THOUGHT FOR TODAY: I will mark my baby's coming with a ritual gesture that expresses my feelings and celebrates the continuity of life.

If I bear burdens

they begin to be remembered
as gifts, goods, a basket

of bread that hurts
my shoulders but closes me

in fragrance. I can
eat as I go.
    —DENISE LEVERTOV

It's easy to forget what a blessing this pregnancy is, as it becomes more of a burden and less of a pleasure. Waiting and anxiety can sap your strength, so that you become cross without meaning to be, as though you were angry with your baby for waiting to be born, for finishing itself off.

In this last month, the baby's body is mainly adding fat, fat that will make it strong and healthy, able to thrive during the hard work of being an infant. After birth, it will have to learn how to take nourishment through its mouth; your baby will have to work for a living, like the rest of us, instead of letting everything flow into it.

You can turn the burden of waiting into a gift, if you remember that every day makes your baby safer, stronger, closer to the person you want to see.

THOUGHT FOR TODAY: I have the power to transform my perception, if I choose, from negative to positive.

Day 11

If one but realized it, with the onset of the first pangs of birth pains, one begins to say farewell to one's baby. For no sooner has it entered the world, when others begin to demand their share. With the child at one's breast, one keeps the warmth of possession a little longer.

—PRINCESS GRACE OF MONACO

I remember feeling after eight months that it was high time other people had a share of my baby. You may feel differently, but I was certainly ready to relinquish "the warmth of possession"; in fact, if I could have detached that baby and let her father carry her around, or her grandparents, that would have been just fine; I didn't insist on single ownership.

Of course, no one will own your baby. And the inevitable struggles in your lives to come will be about control. It's not possession that you'll give up, it's physical connection and interdependence with your baby. That's what will be most difficult for you both, and it's that connection that breast-feeding will keep alive for a bit.

In fact, breast-feeding is the best way for you to learn to separate, because it's a process the baby controls, through the rhythm of its needs. You will come to accept your baby's independence inevitably, as its needs change.

THOUGHT FOR TODAY: My needs and satisfactions and my baby's will be complementary for awhile, and then our relationship will change.

The Ninth Month   267

Day 12

. . . What should we be without
The dolphin's arc, the dove's return,

These things in which we have seen ourselves and spoken?
                                        —RICHARD WILBUR

The rhythm of growth is like an arc: it throws itself forward, then returns near its beginning. We recognize this movement wherever we find it—in the cycle of a flower's growth or in an infant's efforts to be independent: The flower droops toward the earth after blooming, and the infant hastily returns to the safety of mother's or father's arms.

The form pleases us, because it speaks of our own individual rhythms—breathing, heartbeat, the sweetness of solitude and the warmth of homecoming. Your infant will follow this curve, in ways that you may find charming, touching, or exasperating. It will try to move out on its own long before it's ready, and rush back many times.

Every child wants independence, yet every one also longs for security. In our lives many of us recognize these twin desires that impel us out, then back. Both are valuable, and you will learn to help your baby to balance these impulses so its new life will create the most beautiful arc.

THOUGHT FOR TODAY: I am my baby's connection to both physical comfort and spiritual strength, and I will do my best to foster its true independence.

Day 13

Two things in the world you never regret; a swim in the ocean, the birth of a child.

—MARY GORDON

Although childbirth now is far safer than it has ever been in the recorded history of the human species, some aspects of twentieth-century hospital birth procedures may be cruel to infants. Birth produces a trauma, many psychologists feel, so that literally we all regret our births. Much of our energy, according to their theories, is spent seeking conditions that evoke the comfort and security of life in the womb.

Yet babies recover wonderfully from the shocks of their birth and embrace with gusto the adventure of living. Perhaps it's only as grown-ups that we feel this regret. Babies are too busy learning the fascinating puzzles of civilized behavior to long for placental bliss.

As we've said earlier, regret is a sterile, unproductive thing. No matter what our real constraints or shortcomings, life is far too rich to waste time on it. Your baby won't regret its birth, at least not for many years. Concentrating on your blessings will help you to let go of any regrets as well.

THOUGHT FOR TODAY: As an ocean swim invigorates my body, the birth of my baby will refresh my spirit. We have much to teach each other.

> *Is it you? Are you there,*
> *thief I can't see,*
>   *drinking,*
>   *leaving me at the edge*
>   *of breathing?* . . .
>
>   *is it you, penny face?*
>   *Is it you?*
>   —KATHLEEN FRASER

In the last months of pregnancy many women feel the intermittent tightening of the uterus known as Braxton-Hicks contractions. These aren't the contractions of labor—they're almost a practice for it. Sometimes they go away if you move around, but sometimes they don't; I remember having them every night between five and seven o'clock, whether I was standing up, sitting down, or walking around.

Sometimes during a Braxton-Hicks contraction your doctor can actually see your uterus tipping up, as it will during true labor. This can be exciting because any evidence of your baby's presence is exciting in these final weeks and days.

Soon enough your questions will be answered. You'll see the face that has been hidden from eyes until now; your spirit has also prepared a welcome for your guest, and in this recognition there will be no surprise.

THOUGHT FOR TODAY: My baby is at the same time a stranger and totally known. I'm grateful for this opportunity to expand my capacity to love.

Day 15

When we start out, having a baby sounds like undertaking a personal project. But this is not a paint-by-number kit. . . . We act as a conduit for a totally distinct person here.
                                        —ANNA QUINDLEN

Some women say that their first experience of their baby's individuality comes during the birth. They realize that they are not totally in control of what is happening; that even their doctor or nurse is not in total control; another person has entered the picture, someone with her or his own body, needs, and program for development.

The Braxton-Hicks contractions may be signals from that distinct person; they may have to do with your baby's readiness to be born rather than with the condition of your own body. It's often difficult to separate, even in thought, your baby from your pregnancy; yet they're distinct.

You might find it helpful later to begin thinking of your baby as a separate individual now. Parenting will be eased when the boundaries between your child and yourself are firm and secure.

THOUGHT FOR TODAY: For eight and a half months I've been a channel for my baby, but soon I'll welcome her or his individuality.

THIS MONTH'S VISIT TO THE DOCTOR

Date:

Weight: Blood Pressure:

Weight Gain:

Signs of Pregnancy Since Last Visit:

Changes in Eating:

Changes in Sleeping:

Changes in Activities/Energy Level:

Reflections:

Questions for Next Visit:

Day 16

To the rational mind grant
Things rational. But to the spirit
(All things there possible)
Accord what is spiritual.
　　　　　　—RICHARD EBERHART

Even now, you may have fears about your safety, or your baby's. In past times, childbirth was hazardous for many women, and it remains so today for poor women who lack sensitive birth care. But for a well-nourished woman with adequate material resources, the danger is slim.

To your material resources, add the spiritual ones you have been developing over these months. They will sustain you, body and spirit, whatever happens in the coming weeks. Truly, all things are possible to a strong, bright spirit. Acceptance of whatever comes can be eased when you detach from life's details and remind yourself that no one sees the whole picture.

Your rational mind is one of your resources—your curiosity and intelligence have helped you prepare yourself for your child's birth in the best possible way. Combined with help from your birth partners and advisors, and with your shining spirit, it's part of a winning team.

THOUGHT FOR TODAY: I am doing as well as I can the difficult task of both preparing carefully for this birth and detaching from it.

Day 17

This is flesh I'm talking about here. Flesh that needs to be loved. Feet that need to rest and to dance; backs that need support; shoulders that need arms, strong arms I'm telling you.

—TONI MORRISON

Birth is hard work, and your baby will be tuckered out by it. Depending on what kind of an experience you have, you may recover more quickly; your baby's body is smaller and its muscles are less developed, and besides, she or he is also learning to do many strange new independent things, like breathing, sucking, and coping with the pressure of cool, dry air.

The language of loving touch is understood by flesh. Massage is a wonderful way to communicate with your baby; lovingly rubbing its limbs, chest, and back with mild lotion gives the baby feelings of love and pleasure that increase its ability to relax and to trust you.

You may be surprised by the sheer physical pleasure you feel in touching your baby, but this bond is a deep and precious one. Let loving touch awaken your sensitivity to your baby's body; it will nourish you, too.

THOUGHT FOR TODAY: My body and my baby's body will continue to communicate after birth, and I will rejoice in this bond.

Day 18

The leading human trait [is] the attempt to defy the force of gravity. Gravity—we're all trying to beat it all our lives. You can see it in the games we play—jumping, running, tennis. It's an instinct.

—CHRISTINA STEAD

Many authorities have speculated about the role of gravity in the birth process. On the one hand are those who say the mother's position should be as close to upright as possible for the birth, so that gravity can aid the baby's movement through the birth canal, and on the other are those who maintain that any slight advantage this might give is outweighed by the comfort and safety of having the mother lying more or less supine, on her back supported by pillows. In the middle are the proponents of giving birth in a tank of water.

You probably won't have a chance to test different alternatives, for when labor begins usually parents are caught up in the exciting, dynamic process. For this reason, be sure you explore any questions you have with your doctor or midwife well ahead of time. Every birth is different, as every mother and baby are different, and there is no such thing as a perfect solution to any question.

THOUGHT FOR TODAY: Whatever style of birthing I choose, it will be the right one for me.

> *My nipples are cathedrals,*
> *My flesh is a miracle. I flow to the ocean*
> *Where all the rivers of the earth come together.*
> *My body is a holy vessel. I am fire and air.*
> —GRACE SHULMAN

Have you ever seen any of the pieces of needle art that make up the huge art work called "The Birth Project"? Conceptualized and coordinated by artist Judy Chicago and executed by dozens of talented stitchers around the United States and abroad, the work establishes a new series of heroic images of women to set against the heroic male images of classical and modern art.

The birth image central to this work of art celebrates the fertility of the female body and the ordinary heroism of childbirth. Even if you think that a lot of rhetoric glorifying motherhood is soppy or excessive, you may find these images compelling. And even if you never see them, you are taking your place among them. The work celebrates all women, all birth, all giving of life. It's high time women artists developed a language of images to celebrate one of our most profound experiences.

THOUGHT FOR TODAY: I deserve to feel a part of any heroic cultural image of motherhood. My body is strong and willing, and any art that celebrates women's strength affirms me.

Day 20

Life itself is the test and there is no end to the testing as long as the person breathes.

—Murshida Vera Justin Corda

Is my life a test? If so, for what? I prefer to think that I've already passed whatever test there is, with flying colors, and that the experience I'm storing up each day is further evidence of my success.

There's no way you can fail at our joint endeavor. Whatever happens, you are part of the universal pattern of which our daily lives form only a tiny part. Tiny yet essential; every atom is essential to the whole, and the whole resonates and vibrates with the sound and movement of our millions of voices, bodies, lives.

True, life presents us with new challenges. But if we meet them wholeheartedly, we can't fail. You've already succeeded in having the very best pregnancy you could have. Your baby's birth will be another success, no matter what its details are. When you take a broad perspective on your life, you can appreciate how well you are doing.

THOUGHT FOR TODAY: I will let go of any notion that I'm being tested against anyone or anything. I'm tested only in the sense that every day I have a chance to prove my strength.

Day 21

> *But the imagination*
> *knows all stories*
> *before they are told.*
> —WILLIAM CARLOS WILLIAMS

Just as our bodies keep the knowledge of all phases of our growth, so our minds store all the feelings and ideas that accompany them. Our imaginations are rich with possibility; every achievement and every loss in our lives becomes part of our story.

Each of us is individual in the way we interpret our own stories. Not only do similar events hold different meanings for different people, but we can change a story's meaning if it doesn't satisfy us. Death, divorce, miscarriage, all such losses are felt as blows to the self, yet when we tell these stories over to ourselves, we can find great value in survival and in the deepening and softening of our spirits that may follow loss.

You may be feeling impatience or boredom now. Yet in retrospect these last weeks of pregnancy may come to seem valuable in a way you don't imagine. Even if you're in physical discomfort or confined to bed, this is a precious time—your last time before the baby is born, before your questions are answered.

THOUGHT FOR TODAY: Let me find in my imagination today the story that will help me to accept my present reality, and to revel in it.

Day 22

The body goes about its business without our conscious participation. The late night janitorial staff, moving quietly through the building at night, locking windows, sweeping floors, emptying waste baskets, the silent labor necessary for us to go about our everyday preoccupations. And how we hate it when the smoothly working, efficient system breaks down, even for a day.

—MADELON SPRENGNETHER

Some days it may seem that your body's efficient maintenance staff has quit. You may be constipated, and your ankles may swell. Your fingers might feel puffy. Simply getting out of bed in the morning can be an elaborate chore, and finding a comfortable position for sleep is a nightly challenge.

How rare it is to be aware of the body's workings. This is an opportunity for you to tune in more closely to your body's business, the retention and release of fluids, the clearing of breakdown products from muscles and cells. You may never again be at this point of heightened awareness. It isn't merely a negative feature of late pregnancy; it's also a chance for you to appreciate your body's miraculous functioning. Not only is it able to grow and nurture a new life; even when stressed, it continues to perform the ordinary miracles that keep you pulsing, breathing, digesting, and eating.

THOUGHT FOR TODAY: I will turn over my feelings; the bright underside of discomfort is heightened consciousness. My spirit gives thanks for this body.

Day 23

When you begin, begin at the beginning.
Begin with magic, begin with the sun,
Begin with the grass.
—HELEN WOLFERT

"The beginning," as you've come to realize, is a pretty arbitrary description. When did your baby's growth begin—when sperm met ovum, at implantation, or earlier, when your ova matured? Or perhaps it has not yet begun—will you consider birth the real beginning of your face-to-face relationship with the new life?

After your baby's birth you may find yourself involved in more talk about beginnings—where did this or that feature of the child's body or personality come from? "No one in our family ever had straight toes"; "Your side of the family is good at math." Knowing as we do that the strands of nurture and heredity are so entwined that it's not possible to assign human traits definitively to one or the other, you'll be wise to cut such speculation short.

All talk of beginnings leads back to some form of the chicken-and-egg controversy. It might be better to begin with magic, the unknowable. This at least allows us to surrender both our ignorance and our knowledge, to admit we can't understand. The appropriate response is wonder.

THOUGHT FOR TODAY: Through this pregnancy I have developed my sense of the holy to the point where I'm able to be awed by the infinite delicacy of life.

Day 24

As much as anything, being a parent is about loss. Every day you wake up to discover a slightly different person sleeping in that cradle, that crib, that bottom bunk, that dinosaur sleeping bag.

—JOYCE MAYNARD

Certainly, the makers of instant cameras would like us all to think that passing moments are "lost" unless we capture them on expensive film. But our minds' eyes are far more effective cameras. Nothing is ever lost; remember the add-a-pearl necklace? The child sleeping in the crib used to be the baby who slept in the cradle, and that baby survives inside the child. You know it's there, and the child will come to know it in good time.

Memories are rich precisely because they pile on top of one another, like layers of soil, penetrated by the warmth of our love. Sad memories are tempered by the adjacent joys, and past happinesses are a little blurred and softened by our losses.

To the growing spirit, all moments are precious and none is lost. Motherhood is about growing and changing. The two-year-old's mother carries within her the mother of the newborn infant, the pregnant woman, and the young girl, and she knows everything they knew.

THOUGHT FOR TODAY: I too am a slightly different person every day, but this is only a loss if I choose to see it that way.

Day 25

> *You know the water will freeze*
> *then melt, the stone will crack,*
> *even if not in your lifetime.*
> —DEENA LINETT

In the Middle Ages, generations of stonemasons and carvers worked on the great cathedrals, knowing that none of them would see the finished building, yet happy to contribute their skills. Many modern scientists think of their projects in similar terms, as collective endeavors that none of them will live to see "finished."

The great project of changing the world is like this. When we look back over recent centuries we can see much that looks like solid human advancement—yet so much remains to be done. Having this baby is part of your contribution to the future, to the building of a cleaner, more equitable, peaceful world.

Our world is full of uncracked stones. Rather than worrying about them, turn your energies to the care and nurture of your own little drops of water. Each child that's born into a family where love and understanding nurture life can help to change the world for the better.

THOUGHT FOR TODAY: I don't expect any quick payoffs. Caring for ourselves and our families is our best way to care for the world, in the long term.

Day 26

For several generations people have always hoped for "something better" for their children than they had themselves; is that impetus used up?

—CHRISTA WOLF

For most people in the world, the hope of a better life for our children still means a more equal share in society's wealth. For the fortunate few who have achieved a high standard of living, "something better" may be unrealistic, if it's understood merely as more material goods. After all, what can be better than prosperity?

The only thing better than having a fair share of abundance is helping others to share it also. Whether your family is comfortable or just scraping by, you can not only hope for a better life for your child but actively plan for it. You can share with your child the knowledge of how lopsidedly our world's abundance is distributed, and the commitment to even it out.

Some people think societies can grow too fat, corrupted by excesses of material goods and expectations of luxury. There's no such thing as excessive spiritual development, however. Teaching our children to live better—more humanely, more lovingly—with less—consuming less energy, producing less waste—may be the key to a better life for them.

THOUGHT FOR TODAY: The resources of the spirit, unlike those of our environment, are infinitely renewable.

Joy & Woe are woven fine,
A Clothing for the Soul divine;
Under every grief & pine
Runs a joy with silken twine.
　　　　　　　—WILLIAM BLAKE

The final days of pregnancy can be a time of fluctuating feelings, perhaps even more so than the months leading up to them. You may have grown accustomed to rapid changes in your emotional temperature—perhaps starting the day with a high heart only to find yourself struggling later with a fatigue that seems close to despair.

Moments of anguish make our moments of radiance shine all the brighter. Suffering softens our spirits and opens us to joy. We need variation; even unbroken bliss would become monotonous. Let your knowledge of this human rhythm sustain you through your most difficult hours, as you call on your source of never-failing strength.

Many people remember to pray only when they are sad; others only when things are going well. As a wise friend said to me once, "When help seems far away, ask yourself who moved?" This can help you to make a habit of prayer. You'll do well to invest your energy in prayer and meditation; they'll pay a lifetime of dividends.

THOUGHT FOR TODAY: However my life appears to me at this moment, I know one thing for sure: it will change.

Day 28

There are two perfectly good people, one dead and the other unborn.

—CHINESE PROVERB

The unborn soul within you has never made a mistake. Yet. It will start with a clean slate, in a state of perfect goodness, because it is too small and weak to do anything at all, let alone something rotten.

Perfect goodness can't last, however, and it won't be small and weak for very long, either. As soon as your baby is able to act, it will make mistakes. She or he will ruin a perfect record, thereby joining the human race.

Your baby will be perfectly her- or himself, but that's the only kind of perfection any of us ever attains. Perfect goodness is an ideal; we worship as saints those few human beings among us who seem to lead perfect lives, in which they hurt no one and benefit many. Yet even the lives of saints include episodes of doubt, error, impatience, or thoughtlessness. Used properly, the ideal of perfection can guide you as your baby grows up, but it should never become a punishment for either one of you.

THOUGHT FOR TODAY: As I accept my own imperfections, I will accept and love my child's.

Day 29

> *You take high place*
> *as hills take sun—*
> *being inevitably there*
> *in the path of the sun.*
> —LOLA RIDGE

In about a week, you and your baby will be two people. You may have grown so accustomed to thinking of the baby as a part of yourself that it will be odd to find it a distinct person. Of course, you will be tied together for a while, by the baby's need to nurse and your need to nurse it. That bond is a precious one; your baby's hunger and your ability to feed it will give you both an experience of powerful mutual satisfaction.

For the next little while, your baby will definitely take high place. Because it has grown inside your body, your sense of it is a part of your sense of yourself, and you will feel its needs and its helplessness almost as though they were your own. Your spirit will have to give birth to your baby's spirit, just as your body will release its separate body.

When this doesn't happen properly, distorted relationships result. In your family, you can have healthy respect for one another's integrity. There is a spiritual as well as a physical kind of weaning.

THOUGHT FOR TODAY: My partner and I will cherish our baby unconditionally, so that it can grow as an individual according to its own life plan.

Day 30

> *Now this is the day.*
> *Our child,*
> *Into the daylight*
> *You will go out standing.*
> *Preparing for your day,*
> *We have passed our days.*
> —Zuni prayer

You have passed a lot of days preparing for your baby's day. You may have gone through a nesting phase, when you painted and scraped and shopped and sewed and ironed so that your baby's space would be welcoming. You may have spent hundreds of hours working on your body, learning to lift your abdomen with breaths so as to ease your baby's birth, creaming your skin so it will be soft and flexible, massaging your nipples so they won't crack when your child nurses. You have nourished the two of you as best you could, swallowing everything you could stand to swallow that would do you good, and rigorously abstaining from things that wouldn't. At times, you may be tempted to challenge your baby, at least in your thoughts: "See, I've done all this. Now, it's up to you."

In your case, challenge is irrelevant. The best condition for your baby's growth is your unconditional love and acceptance. Beyond that, it's out of your hands.

THOUGHT FOR TODAY: I give thanks for my days of preparation, and I pray for the serenity to greet my baby with an open heart.

Help us to be the always hopeful
Gardeners of the spirit
Who know that without darkness

Nothing comes to birth
As without light
Nothing flowers
—MAY SARTON

Because you are a human being and not a character in a story or a cutout paper doll, nothing in your life will ever be unmixed. At your most exquisite peak moments you may feel twinges of disappointment, panic, or absurd hilarity. And when you are saddest, most hopeless, you usually can find a space for a healthy spark of anger or humor.

For all its solemnity, birth is also a mixed experience. Many women say it was harder work than they ever knew they were capable of, but occasionally a woman is surprised by how easy her labor seems. Some women have strong sexual feelings during the process, while others can't imagine anything further from an erotic activity.

All you can be sure of is that your birth experience will be unique. It's likely that you'll have some mixed feelings; that it won't be what you expected; and that the outcome will be a healthy baby. A higher power accompanies you in labor and delivery, as it has throughout pregnancy.

THOUGHT FOR TODAY: Without darkness, I can't perceive light. I'm grateful for the variety of my experience.

THIS MONTH'S VISIT TO THE DOCTOR

Date:

Weight: Blood Pressure:

Weight Gain:

Signs of Pregnancy Since Last Visit:

Changes in Eating:

Changes in Sleeping:

Changes in Activities/Energy Level:

Reflections:

First Day Past Due Date

We have discovered today that the stimulus that sets labor in motion comes from the child, just as the Ancients said it did. And now we know that the child actually does struggle to be born.

—FREDERICK LEBOYER

Oh, for heaven's sake; here's your first date with your new baby, and it's late. What kind of a relationship is this going to be? Can't the baby tell you're nearly jumping out of your skin with anticipation—bouncing off the walls in eagerness? Maybe something's wrong.

Most likely, nothing is wrong. Your baby too is waiting for a signal, from some source beyond control. Billions of babies have been born, very few of them at will. What you need, right now, is serenity.

You probably wish your child would start struggling to be born, anything to break the calm. Yet you know that in this process, as in all the most important things in life, you must surrender your will, set your ego and its expectations on one side, and turn over the process to the power of life itself. Your long wait will end; you are in good hands.

THOUGHT FOR TODAY: My regular practice of meditation and prayer has strengthened my spirit. I'm grateful for the exercise.

290

Second Day Past Due Date

I have wandered over the fruitful earth
But I never came here before,
Oh, lift me over the threshold, and let me in at the door!
　　　　　　　　　—MARY ELIZABETH COLERIDGE

When the real right time comes for your baby to be born, all doubts will be gone. It needs to enter this world every bit as much as you need to let it go. This birthing will be a mutual process.

More than just you and your baby are involved. The great forces that human beings have always feared and worshiped are very close to you now, the gods of creation and destruction, of the great cycle of life with all its changes.

In some faiths, newborn babies are believed to carry souls that have lived before, in other bodies. According to this belief, your spirit might be specifically immortal; you might have lived before, in China, Peru, Africa, or Alaska, and so might your baby. The wheel of time has brought you into intimate relation now, and your destinies will be fulfilled.

THOUGHT FOR TODAY: The immortality of the spirit is no more miraculous than the creation and growth of a new life within me. I accept all miracles.

Third Day Past Due Date

Labor is blossoming or dancing
Where body is not bruised to pleasure soul.
—W. B. YEATS

In earlier centuries, many mothers' and babies' lives were lost because of conditions that can now be dealt with fairly simply. Hospitals now have all sorts of machines for intervening in the progress of human birthing, and often they are very good things indeed. One woman's baby simply didn't want to be born; three weeks after the due date her obstetrician induced labor, and a healthy infant was born four hours later, with fingernails grown far past the ends of its tiny fingers.

Intervention was appropriate in this case—although there will be times when midwives and doctors disagree on the best way to trigger the release of oxytocin, the hormone that initiates labor.

You are fortunate, because you have both a healthy, well-prepared body and skilled support systems. Your labor will be both a dance and a blossoming.

THOUGHT FOR TODAY: I can trust myself to know what my baby and I need, from the great array of technology that's available.

Fourth Day Past Due Date

In the beginning, the Greeks said, there was only formless chaos: light and dark, sea and land, blended in a shapeless pudding. Then chaos settled into form, and that form was the huge Gaea, the deep-breasted one, the earth. In the timeless span before creation, she existed to herself and of herself alone.

—PATRICIA MONAGHAN

The work of creation is done; chaos long ago settled into form, and that form is now occupying you. However much you may feel like a shapeless pudding, you know that within a few days, most likely, you'll give birth to the new life.

This is your last chance to exist to yourself and of yourself alone for quite a while. Can you detach from your eagerness enough to enjoy yourself? A manicure, a pedicure, a morning spent writing in your journal—these will become rare luxuries after the baby is born.

You and your partner can use this little bit of time to renew your intimacy. Many relationships fray under the stress of late pregnancy and the first weeks postpartum. Give yourself a treat; use this unexpected time creatively. You probably don't want to go white-water canoeing or downhill skiing, but a whirlpool bath or a drive in the country are within reach.

THOUGHT FOR TODAY: All time is a gift. If I can accept that, I can take pleasure in these days.

Fifth Day Past Due Date

The pears are all gone from the tree but I imagine them hanging there, ripe curves within the many scimitar leaves, and within them many pears of the coming season. I feel like a pear. I hang secret within the curling leaves, just as the pear would be hanging on its tree.

—MERIDEL LeSUEUR

Your energies are focused on the coming birth, and you will need them for the momentous events of labor, delivery, nursing, and new parenthood. This is not the end of a process, however, but the beginning of a new phase in your life. When the pear tree yields up its fruit, it can stand dormant until the next season. Human parenthood involves a little more continuous responsibility; human fruit must be fed and diapered, washed and rocked, immunized, trained, and educated. No doubt that's why most human families are so small, at least compared to pear trees.

You may repeat this process several times. Each pregnancy and birth will be unique, though after the first some of the sense of adventure may be gone. Your body does resemble a ripe pear in its fullness and solidity, but the only secret that remains is your baby. In these last days of pregnancy perhaps your child is growing sweeter, like a late pear.

THOUGHT FOR TODAY: My body is capable of many ripenings, and so is my spirit.

Sixth Day Past Due Date

With the ground plowed, we
carried buckets of water to soak the earth.
Seeds hugged themselves below, cleaving
to the lime and foam.
—ROBYN WIEGMAN

Does it feel to you as though your baby is hugging itself below, cleaving to you as seeds cling to the earth? Before the powerful force of labor begins to summon it, the baby is closed within your body and you can't imagine, if you haven't already given birth, how it will be dislodged. You may also have anxieties about the pain and effort of labor and delivery.

Your fear, if you feel it, is natural—this is a major life event you're anticipating, and literature and folklore have richly embroidered it. Hold on to what you have learned about the birth process, and trust in your partner, your doctor, your midwife, yourself.

Sometimes a pregnant woman fantasizes that her fear may be holding back her baby's birth; it isn't. Babies are born as surely as seeds burst and shoots break ground. Your baby is obeying its own internal timetable, the same one that will determine the pace of its growth. Your task is to cooperate with the burgeoning seed.

THOUGHT FOR TODAY: Once I accept it as natural, I can let go of my fear and let it flow through me. New feelings will come in its place.

Seventh Day Past Due Date

. . . the pains of childbirth were altogether different from the enveloping effects of other kinds of pain. These were pains one could follow with one's mind. . . .

—MARGARET MEAD

In almost every woman's labor there comes a point when she is so deeply involved in the effort that rational thought or commentary isn't possible. Until that point, though, many women say they can actively feel the stretching of their cervical opening and the pressure of the contracting womb on the baby's body.

Life doesn't deal us more than we can handle. Most labors begin gradually and build in intensity over four to sixteen hours. The average length of first labors is about twelve hours, but for most of this time, contractions usually are light. If you look at labor and delivery as opportunities for learning basic facts about your own body, you're bound to have an interesting time.

THOUGHT FOR TODAY: I know I have little to fear from the coming birth, and a new life to gain.

Eighth Day Past Due Date

Now even as the world descends
My mother my mold my maker
Is with me to the end.
　　　　—Patricia Goedicke

In our culture it's not usual for mothers to attend their daughters' labor and delivery, though in many cultures it's a valued part of the mother-daughter relationship. Some women like to have women friends in attendance when they give birth. Whoever is going to be with you during labor— partner, midwife, or other coach—needs to understand what you want. Since your attention is going to be focused more on your process than on communication, this birth attendant should be someone with whom you have a comfortable level of intimacy.

The muscles that move in the birth process are seldom felt at any other time. Some women say labor and birth seem cosmic; their contractions feel vast as earthquakes and the baby's head emerges with the force of a mountain. Any attendants who are with you will share in your awe.

THOUGHT FOR TODAY: I will be quite selfish in my choice of birth attendants, for I deserve all possible comfort and support.

Ninth Day Past Due Date

Nature demands a certain devotion, and she demands a period of struggling with her.

—VINCENT VAN GOGH

Artists must struggle to find the means within themselves to reflect what they want to express. In labor and delivery, the expression happens without your individual decision—though not always without a struggle. Every birth is a passionately exciting drama, starring the mother, designed and stage-managed by her doctor or midwife, and scripted by human evolution.

Scientific ingenuity has managed to give you and your doctor some choices about what happens during the process, but the power of nature is still in control. Your patience and detachment now will help you to accept this power and to cooperate with it. It's important to keep up your practice of breathing and meditation. Nothing has stopped; you're entering the birth process even though it may be slower than your rehearsals.

THOUGHT FOR TODAY: Serenity depends on my accepting the collaboration of forces I can't see or control. I'm grateful for the spiritual discipline that helps me do this.

Tenth Day Past Due Date

There are times when
I think only of how to do away
With this brute power
That cannot be tamed.
                                    —MAY SARTON

Now at last you have discovered the secret of slowing down time: carrying a pregnancy past the due date. Many first-time mothers are positive their babies are going to come early; they feel sure they have set the date of conception too late. Every moment it is possible to feel your body clenching in fear—what if something is wrong?—and to let it go. However tired you may be of lugging your baby around, there is not much you can do about it at this point.

Your baby doesn't move so much these days, but that's because it has grown to fill up all the space in your womb. It has no room for thrashing around, as it did a few months ago. "This brute power" that governs both your lives will soon make itself felt. Meanwhile, you can snatch a little serenity for yourself and your baby by remembering that your source of spiritual strength is constantly available, for you and your partner, with a boundless supply of love and assurance.

THOUGHT FOR TODAY: I pray for the serenity to accept what I cannot change, the courage to change the things I can, and the wisdom to know the difference.

Author Index

Aeschylus, 100
Akhmadulina, Bella, 227
Alta, 175
Angelou, Maya, 257
Anonymous, 111
Anonymous (African American Gospel song), 225
Anonymous (Babylonian myth), 159
Anonymous (Chinese proverb), 285
Anonymous (Gaelic Welcome to the Moon), 9
Anonymous (Inuit song), 121
Anonymous (Navaho lullaby), 166
Anonymous (Seminole song), 61
Anonymous (Zuni prayer), 287
Arendt, Hannah, 201
Atwood, Margaret, 142
Auden, W.H., 229

Bambara, Toni Cade, 62
Barba, Sharon, 36
Benét, William Rose, 255
Berger, John, 74
Bernikow, Louise, 84
Biller, Matthew, 222
Bishop, Elizabeth, 135, 150
Blackwell, Elizabeth, 75, 139
Blake, William, 284
Bly, Carol, 183
Bradstreet, Anne, 68
Brain, Robert, 47
Branch, Anna Hempstead, 17, 43
Brontë, Charlotte, 141, 194
Brontë, Emily, 27, 116, 132